COPING
WITHOUT A CURE

Living with chronic back pain

& Fibromyalgia

AMY SAMUEL

© Amy Samuel (Haskins) 2017

All rights reserved.

No part of this publication may be reproduced or transmitted in any form by any means, electronic or mechanical, including photocopy, recording or any information storage and retrieval system, without permission in writing from the publisher.

Printed by Createspace, an Amazon.com Company.

Published By Amy Haskins.
76 California Rd, Bristol, BS30 9XW, UK.
Email: hippy_amyjo@hotmail.com

Book design by Nathalia Harris.
Word art by Nathalia Harris.
Artwork by Amy Samuel (Haskins).

Scripture references taken from the Holy Bible, New Living Translation (NLT), copyright © 1996, 2004, 2007 by Tyndale House Foundation. Used by permission of Tyndale House Publishers, Inc., Carol Stream, IL 60188. All rights reserved.
And the Holy Bible, the New Internation Version® (NIV®) copyright © 1973, 1978, 1984, 2011 by Biblica, Inc.™ Used by permission. All rights reserved worldwide.

ISBN 978-1547194810

First edition 2017

CONTENTS

Forward	7
Acknowledgements	9
Introduction	11
Section 1 - A Western Medical Approach to Treatment	15
1 Pharmaceutical Medications	16
2 Physiotherapy	23
3 Exercise – Movement as Medicine	27
4 Pain Clinics	47
Section 2 - Alternative Therapies	50
5 Physical Manipulation Therapies	51
6 Massage	57
7 Acupuncture	61
8 Other Therapies I Have Tried	65
9 Magnetic Therapy	69
10 Considering the Spiritual Implications of Alternative Therapies	71
Section 3 - More Practical Self Management	77
11 Nutrition and Supplements	78
12 Sleep	92
13 Other Devices	94
14 Pregnancy and Childbirth	98

Section 4 - Coping Mentally, Emotionally And Spiritually   103
    15 The Neurochemical Link   104
    16 The Power of Positive Thought   108
    17 Creativity and Health   113
    18 Spirituality, and Christian Prayer for Healing   123

Summary   131

Epilogue   135

Bibliography   136

FORWARD

Firstly let me say that I am not a medical professional. I had always wanted to work in medicine or alternative therapy of some kind; the human body has always fascinated me; Health and nutrition fascinate me. We are truly complex and amazing creations and are forever on a journey of discovering more about how to function optimally.

I am writing this book as a sufferer of chronic back pain and fibromyalgia, and as someone who has experience in learning to manage it, or on some days – not manage it! The only way I can sit here writing for an hour or so is because I have already done my stretches, taken my medication, walked a little, applied heat to my back, found a suitable seat and back support, and attached the tens machine for the day.

My aim here is to help other sufferers or their friends/family in understanding and dealing with chronic pain. The word "chronic" often has to be explained. It does not mean severe, though many chronic conditions can be serious. No, "chronic", means persistent over time, enduring, constant. Diabetes is a chronic condition, but chicken pox is not.

Today we live in a society that expects most illnesses to be fixed by modern medicine. Science has evolved so much that a cure is often available, if not, a pill to manage the condition. Therefore chronic conditions, like back pain, fibromyalgia, M.E. Lupus, and others, are misunderstood and hard for people to accept as things that one has to 'live with'. They can either cause or co-exist with a sense of hopelessness, or depression. A person's outlook on life can have an impact on the physical body, and so I approach this book fully aware that the reader needs to consider their mental, emotional, and spiritual health as much as the physical.

More knowledge about health conditions, and the many options for treatment in this day and age, can in itself produce anxiety and stress - we want to choose the right therapy, decide what to spend our money on, and bear in mind what background and verified evidence is behind a therapy. You should consult your own GP or other medical professionals before taking on any of my advice.

Back pain is a major factor that can affect the management of fibromyalgia or similar conditions, and may be a pre-existing or co-existing pain problem. In my case, the back pain led to chronic back pain which led to fibromyalgia as well. Back pain may be due to poor posture, a past injury, occupational strain, or arthritis... this list of possibly causes is extensive and each individual should have their back pain examined and investigated by different professionals to try and get to the root of the problem, if possible. But for me, pain management for both fibromyalgia and back pain is a daily discipline.

I write this book to try and help you on your journey towards managing pain and living life to the fullness of all you can.

ACKNOWLEDGEMENTS

I want to thank my Mum and Dad, for bringing me up with good moral standards and work ethics, and teaching me to be self-disciplined and conscientious, as well as praying about all things and depending on God, especially in circumstances we don't understand. Thank you to those who have read drafts and contributed to the content or design of this book – Jess Mountifield, Nathalia Harris - who worked on the design, format and publishing of this book, and Pilates teacher Sarah Lloyd-Clarey.

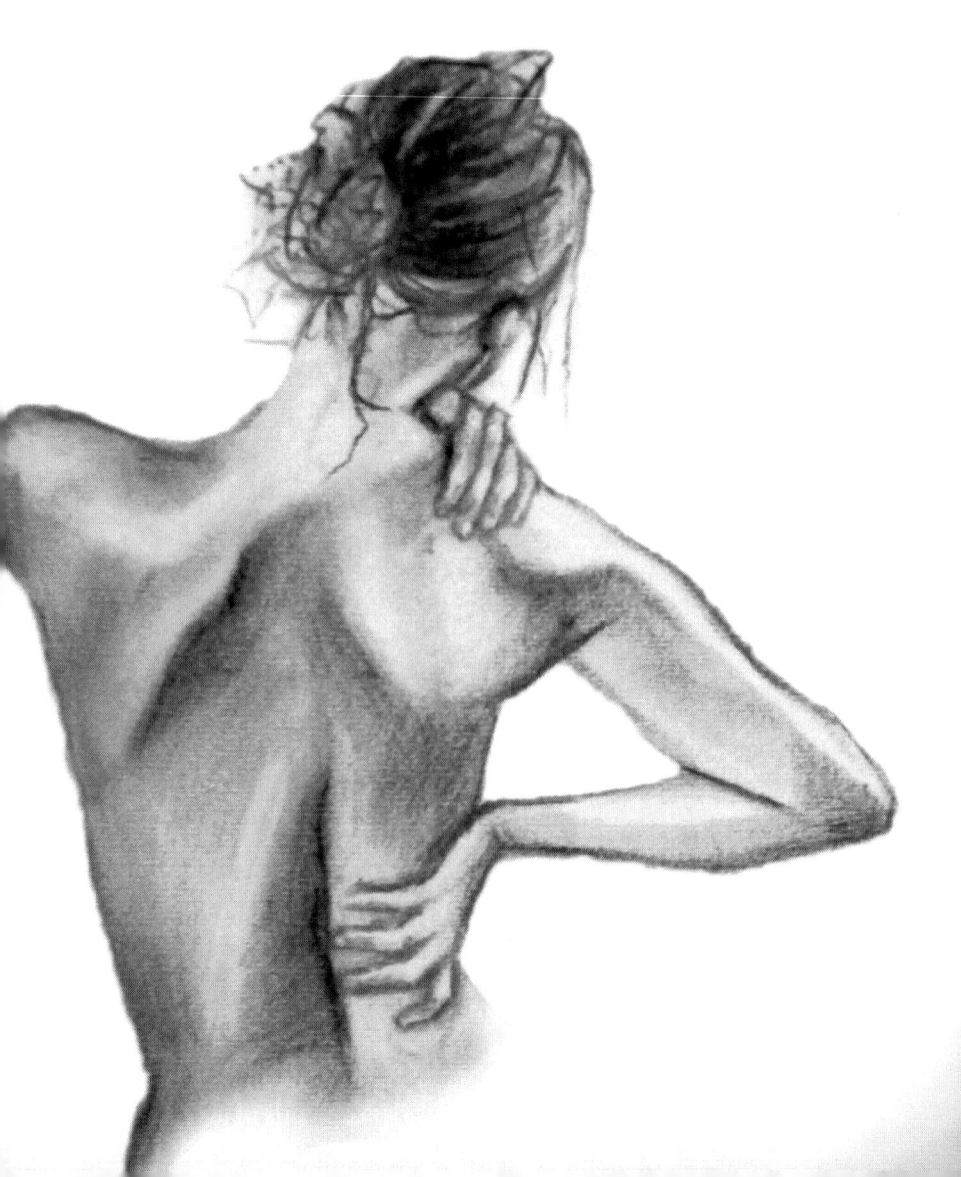

INTRODUCTION

My Story

I will start at the beginning of my journey with pain.

I was 18. Ambitious, worked hard, laziness was the biggest sin, grew up as an active and strong farmer's daughter, and had no problem sitting for hours as I studied through my teens and college. However, working long hours as a waitress and chamber maid, carrying heavy dinner trays with which I then bent over tables, and lifting mattresses to fold the sheets under. I started to have lower back pain. It became a daily thing. And it never went away.

In the first two years of this I visited the GP several times, was given painkillers and referred for physiotherapy. They gave me basic back stretches to do.

I spent countless amounts on chiropractors, osteopaths, osteomyologists, etc. The pain would usually be a lot worse after the chiropractor treatment for a few days and I was told to use ice to recover, then after I would sometimes think it was better for a few days... It wasn't really a consistent reaction.

I of course had to give up work, but continued to push myself through college, which was hard. I frequently held back the tears on the bus because sitting was so painful, just until I could get somewhere where it wasn't embarrassing. Reading over past diary entries, I find numerous accounts I had written about the daily battle to get up and get motivated, fight pain, try to do life, and overcome days when I felt quite frankly, depressed.

I did do things that helped me keep going in those years - stretches, gentle swimming, visiting a hot tub or sauna, having

Artwork, 'Back & Shoulder' by Amy Jo Haskins (Samuel). Graphite & Charcoal. 2017 www.amyjo-arts.co.uk

a massage when I could afford it, and visits to more gentle osteopaths or craniosacral practitioners.

At age 20 I took a big step and travelled to study music and art in Idaho, USA, where I was led to believe I might find healing amongst the professionals and also Christian healing prayer rooms over there. I will talk more about treatments I tried whilst there later.

Two years later I came home, still in as much pain. But by this time I also had *a lot* of upper back pain and muscle spasms in my neck and shoulders. The GPs proceeded to try out another chain of medications.

With these, and frequent massage, acupuncture, gentle exercise, etc., I fumbled my way through an art degree and work on the side. It was during this time (2008) that my new GP diagnosed me with fibromyalgia, which in those days was virtually unknown.

Some years later, in 2013, I finally convinced a top spinal surgeon to perform what might have been a life changing operation, a '*cure*' that I had searched for, for so many years.

MRI scans had already shown that my inter-vertebral discs at L4 and L5 were dehydrated (showing up as dark on the scan, as opposed to light/white, which are the ones which have fluid in). This caused the vertebrae to rub against each other over the years. However years earlier consultants had told me that even people who experience no pain have dehydrated discs and they could not do anything for me, and that I should carry on living with the pain and learn to manage it as best I could. That was around 2002. By 2012 the new scans showed the same condition, but on a CT scan this surgeon could also see a crack in the vertebrae. He proposed to fix and fuse this crack and the disks that were bothering me, including borrowing some bone from my hip to put back into my spine.

He did not promise a miracle, but I believed in one! In fact he was also hesitant to operate on me because of the risks, but I made the decision to have the operation. I went through the procedure, followed by around 6 month's bed-rest with careful physiotherapy.

Yet today, (3 ½ years later) I am still battling pain on a mostly daily basis. But now I have more in my hips and that limits my ability to exercise. Why, we aren't sure.

Some days it brings me to tears, and I take extra medication or might have an extra glass of wine! But most of the time, I cope. I manage pain. This book is about how, and maybe it can encourage you. Or at least know that someone else can understand some of your battle. Being misunderstood is a major disadvantage to those of us with invisible illnesses, especially those that vary from day to day and hour to hour. People who don't see you every day can't understand why on some days you can walk three miles, but can barely walk across the car park on other days.

If you are suffering one of these diseases and reading this book, you are probably looking for a deeper understanding, for answers, for a cure. I would love to give that to you, but it will be more about empowering you to make decisions, and think in helpful ways, to manage your condition in the best way you can.

God grant me the *Serenity* to accept the things I cannot change, courage to *change* the things I can & *wisdom* to know the difference.

THE SERENITY PRAYER

SECTION I

A Western Medical Approach To Treatment

I have tried to divide this section on treatments between western medicine and *'alternative'* medicine, for the sake of structure, however they do not always oppose each other – they are increasingly being used in tandem in the treatment of illness, and I certainly use them in combination. So there will be some over-laps in content. An increasing number of medical doctors and people such as physiotherapists are recognizing the benefits of both approaches, and advising a more holistic, integrative approach to treatment. There are many *'alternative'* therapies that remain misunderstood by scientific testing and mainstream medicine, and so they are not available or recommended on, say, the NHS in the UK. Although conventional medicine seeks an understanding of how treatments actually work, it is not legitimate to exclude treatments which have been shown to work just because we do not understand how. I will discuss in this book those alternative therapies if which I have had some experience, but this is not an exhaustive study on the many treatments on offer which could be helpful or unhelpful.

CHAPTER 1:

Pharmaceutical Medications

I have of course trialled lots of medications for pain relief over the years. I will give a basic description of how they work and my experience of using them – though of course every individual is different, and a person's metabolism can even affect how well a drug may work. Also none of them should be tried without the prescribing and supervision of a doctor. If you feel you have already exhausted the options of prescribed medication for you and are not interested in trying any more, then please skip this chapter!

NSAIDS

The first type of painkiller the GP's will prescribe is a general anti-inflammatory – typically non-steroidal anti-inflammatory drugs (NSAIDS). They are typically used for aches and pains, headaches, flu, period pain, etc., and are available as tablets or in some cases, creams that can be applied directly to the affected area. Ibuprofen can be bought over the counter, but others need a prescription. Examples that I have tried include naproxen, diclofenac, and mefanamic acid. These were tried in the first few years of back pain, and I thought that they bought some relief, but for some reason the effects wore off after a few months of taking them regularly. Aside from that, they can cause side effects such as digestive problems, stomach ulcers, which did affect me, and so the general practice is then to prescribe something like omeprazole alongside them to combat the stomach ulcer. Omeprazole belongs to group of drugs called proton pump inhibitors. It decreases the amount of acid produced in the stomach.

For those for whom anti-inflammatorys are unsuitable, basic paracetamol may be effective. I have never found it to be so, but certainly it is for some people and is quite safe if taken in the recommended dosage.

NARCOTICS

Failing those above options, a narcotic may be prescribed. These are also known as opioids. Examples of opioids include codeine, morphine, tramadol, Fentanyl (which is applied to the skin as a patch, rather than a tablet). Opioids are used for acute pain or after surgery for short term recovery, as well as in long-term pain management. Opinions and experiences of their use in long-term conditions are controversial and differ from person to person. Personally I have found only codeine (or dihydrocodeine has also been prescribed for me, but I found no difference) helpful in managing my condition, but not without experiencing unpleasant side effects.

Common codeine side effects include:
feeling dizzy or drowsy;
nausea, vomiting, stomach pain;
constipation;
sweating; or
mild itching or rash.

I can experience all of the above side effects, but also a numbed/low mood, extreme tiredness, and virtually non-existent libido (though that could be due to other medications I take as well). That said, without pain relief when I really need it, I could not do gentle exercise, which is essential in pain management, and also daily function to teach piano lessons, be a mother, do the house work, even sit to do therapeutic craft-making, etc.... all of which are crucial to me managing chronic pain and low mood. It's a daily thing to decide whether the pain and limitation would be worse than the side effects, if I don't take the medication.

Also, taking more than prescribed is obviously not recommended – one reason being, as with all drugs in my experience, the more you take, the more tolerant your body becomes and you need more to have a pain relieving effect. On 'good' days, I take a break from codeine.

To combat the nausea associated with continued use of these medications, I was prescribed an anti-sickness tablet called cyclyzine. However I understand this cannot be taken in pregnancy, and also induced more tiredness.

To combat the digestive problems, I have found over-the-counter alternative supplements the most helpful, and also good for general digestive health. Peppermint oil capsules are wonderful to help with uncomfortable indigestion, if taken with a meal – rather than chewing lots of chalky antacids! And I absolutely swear by probiotics for healthy digestion (see section on nutritional supplements).

Since I have been taking codeine for years I don't suffer much with constipation now, but it is a very common side effect for most people and certainly was in the first years of taking it. Laxatives may be taken under the direction of your GP, but I preferred to just ensure I ate a high fibre diet, including plenty of dried apricots, prunes, linseeds, and sweet corn!

As far as other opioids go, you may try them under the supervision of a GP and see what your experience is. Tramadol never worked for me but does for many people. Morphine and oromorph were prescribed, and absolutely helpful, for me straight after having major back surgery, but ineffective after a few weeks. And for me they had unpleasant side effects.

ANTI-EPILEPTICS
The next category of medications I will talk about are GABA analogues - generally used to treat epilepsy – anti-epileptics, or anti-convulsants. GABA stands for Gamma-Aminubutyric Acid which is an inhibitory neurotransmitter in the body.

A common example is Gabapentin - which affects chemicals and nerves in the body that are involved in the cause of seizures and some types of pain. In recent years, it has been prescribed to those with nerve pain, neuralgia, fibromyalgia, restless leg syndrome, and even other conditions such as bi-polar disorder.

Drugs such as gabapentin, pregabalin, neurontin, work by interfering with the way pain signals are interpreted in the brain and nervous system.

I was prescribed a high dose of these for a number of years, after attending the pain clinic and also being diagnosed with fibromyalgia. I believe they helped, when I think of the activity I was keeping up at that time of my life, compared with now (when I am not taking them). However it is difficult to judge, because I stopped taking them at the same time as having back surgery and other factors are involved. And I still needed narcotic pain relief and all the other pain managing strategies while I was taking them. I would say it is worth trying them if your health professional thinks they may help you, but be aware of side effects.

I was more fatigued whilst taking them, and had poor memory and concentration. If I forgot to take a dose, (or thought I had taken it but hadn't!) or went away and forgot to pack them – I experienced extreme sleepiness, numbness in my limbs and thoughts, and collapsed. Do not forget to take them regularly if you are prescribed them, and detox from them slowly. Also, when I stopped them I dropped in weight, which suggests they may have been unhelpful in managing weight problems. My father is currently on a high dose of pregabalin for neuralgia pain and Parkinson's, and although he has always been overweight, finds it even harder to lose weight now, and needs to sleep a lot.

ANTIDEPRESSANTS AMITRYPTALINE, FLUOXETINE, SEROXAT, CYCLIZINE

Chronic pain and depression are conditions whose symptoms commonly overlap.[1]

Fibromyalgia in particular, is a musculoskeletal condition characterized by widespread pain and muscle tenderness that is often accompanied by fatigue, sleep disturbances, and depression. Therefore antidepressants have been used in the treatment of this type of condition. A low dose of amitryptyline is often prescribed – this belongs to the family of antidepressants called trycyclics (TCAs). My own experience of trying amitryptyline was that it did not help the pain, caused severe depression and suicidal thoughts, and weight gain! But obviously it has been shown to help some people. Duloxetine and

---

1. Much more detailed studies of the links between depression and chronic pain, and their treatments with antidepressant drugs, can be found online... for example 'The use of Antidepressants for Chronic pain' from www.medscape.com/viewarticle/704975

other SSRIs have also been shown effective.

A low level of antidepressant drug is a commonly suggested by a GP for chronic pain conditions. It will be up to the patient if they want to go down this route, as with all drugs, there can be side effects. If low mood or depression preceded the pain condition, or now exists as a result of it, they may be helpful. Personally I have tried various antidepressants but have now been on fluoxetine for many years and found it effective in not only reducing muscle spasms and anxiety, but the low mood that can accompany a life battling pain. Not taking them is not an option for me (having tried to detox and come off them carefully 5 times before!)

In fact, a more positive mood can help one be motivated to do the things that you need to in managing pain – like exercising, socializing, or engaging in other therapeutic activities. And I do not seem to experience any unpleasant side effects from this drug, although everyone is different.

Fluoxetine belongs to a family of drugs called SSRI's – selective serotonin reuptake inhibitors. They are usually the first type of antidepressant prescribed for depression, because they have relatively few side effects. Some other examples include citalopram, paroxetine, and sertraline.

How do they work?

'It's thought that SSRIs work by increasing serotonin levels in the brain. Serotonin is a neurotransmitter (a messenger chemical that carries signals between nerve cells in the brain). It's thought to have a good influence on mood, emotion and sleep.

After carrying a message, serotonin is usually reabsorbed by the nerve cells (known as "reuptake"). SSRIs work by blocking ("inhibiting") reuptake, meaning more serotonin is available to pass further messages between nearby nerve cells.

It would be too simplistic to say that depression and related mental health conditions are caused by low serotonin levels, but a rise in serotonin levels can improve symptoms and make people more responsive to other types of treatment, such as CBT'.

It is worth mentioning here that CBT forms a part of the pain clinic program that is offered on the NHS to those in chronic pain – our thought patterns do in fact have an impact on our physical health and symptoms of pain, and CBT is not just helpful for those with a mentally related illness or addiction. I have been through a few periods of receiving CBT in the past 12 years and always found it helpful.

Pain management requires a holistic approach – treating mind, body and soul – a theme which I will keep reiterating.

MUSCLE RELAXANTS

Muscle relaxants work by doing exactly as they are called – relaxing muscles! A lot of my pain is called by tight muscles and muscle spasms, so I found that anything that physically relaxes me helps. Massage has been the most effective treatment for this, and I will talk about other natural therapies later on.

Whilst living in the States, I was prescribed Carisoprodol, or 'Soma' and these worked wonderfully! Although they are not intended to be prescribed long term because they have an addictive effect - as in the more you take, the more you need for them to work. They can make you feel slightly 'drunk' and so relaxed that inhibitions or concentration can be reduced. I believe that for this reason, and also because they were expensive, they have been taken off the general market and cannot be prescribed any more, at least in the UK and States. I really did struggle when this happened. Other muscle relaxants were tried on me by the GP, but unfortunately most of them were ineffective. They also make you very sleepy. Now I am prescribed diazepam, or 'valium' for acute muscle spasms that I can't seem to deal with in another way, but I am only allowed to take them occasionally, as these can also be addictive. If you experience episodes of acute muscle spasm, you may want to talk to your doctor about trying

2. www.nhs.uk/conditions/SSRIs-(selective-serotonin-reuptake-inhibitors) / Pages/Introduction.aspx

a relaxing medication, or prefer to deal with it naturally, thereby avoiding side effects and other health complications.

Recently there was a very interesting series on the BBC called *'The doctor who gave up drugs'*, presented by Dr Chris van Tulleken, who conducted a social experiment by taking over part of GP surgery and stopping some of the patient's prescription pills, instead getting them to practice non chemical treatments, such as specific exercise. If you would like to found out more, I believe it is available for purchase from the BBC website.

CAPSAICIN CREAM

Although this is not a *'pill'* as with the other medications I describe here, I was prescribed this very recently by my GP to try out on my back pain and any areas of muscle spasm. It is relatively new as a treatment prescribed on the NHS and comes in the form of a cream.

Capsaicin is derived from red chillies. When nerve endings come into contact with capsaicin they produce Substance-P which is a neurotransmitter that carries pain messages to the brain. Apparently, the more the capsaicin is applied, the fewer pain messages are sent to the brain. The cream causes a warm or burning sensation which is said to decrease the longer it is used - I found the sensation unbearably hot and itchy, which prevented me sleeping, so have only used it the once! Perhaps I should give it more chance, and not at bedtime.

CHAPTER 2:

Physiotherapy

If you go to the GP with any back pain or musculoskeletal problem they will usually refer you to physiotherapy as a first port of call. This is available on the NHS and physiotherapists will assess you and then generally teach you how to do appropriate exercises for your problem areas. This topic is so important and extensive that it requires a separate chapter, so please see *'Exercise – Movement as Medicine'* for more information.

HYDROTHERAPY

Physiotherapists may also offer hydrotherapy (exercise sessions in warm water if they have the facilities), or depending on their training, can also offer some sessions of medical acupuncture, infra-red lamp treatments, supports that you can wear, or some have been known to massage or use the Bowen technique. I have experienced all of these from NHS practitioners, and for me, the only effective treatment they offered was hydrotherapy. Other therapies have proved hugely helpful for me, but only by private more highly trained practitioners. (See my sections on acupuncture and massage).

In this topic of hydrotherapy you may also include the use of ice and heat to treat muscular pain, which is endorsed by many physiotherapists but is also a basic treatment you should use at home.

Hot or cold therapy is used in many musculoskeletal conditions to relieve pain. Coldness can reduce swelling and inflammation, and heat can allow more blood (and therefore nutrients) to flow to the tissues and relax the muscles.

The use of regular hot showers or warm baths is probably something you are already doing at home to help the pain. Lovingly massaging creams into your body afterwards can also help, or if a muscle feels inflamed/over worked - the application of ice might be better. I have always had a soft ice pack that can be kept in the fridge or freezer and applied to the area of pain (generally I use this on my lower back) when I feel the pain is due to over-exertion or inflammation. It is advisable to apply cold for only 10-20 minutes, and then re-apply in about an hour.

I use heat more often, because of frequent muscle spasms, or tight muscles. This type of pain is different to the pain I experience when I *'overdo it'*, and I hope you can tell the difference in your own body too. There are a few options and ways to apply heat packs to your body:

•Purchase a wheat bag, which can either be a rectangle shape or be more contoured to go around your neck and shoulders. These are microwaved to the desired temperature before putting on your skin or over your clothing. Amazon stock them at competitive prices, or a good chemist sometimes sell them.

•Single use stick on heat patches can be purchased from chemists and also Amazon, that you either apply directly to the skin or to the inside of your clothes (read the instructions). They can last 8 – 16 hours and are great if you are moving around and can't carry a wheat bag with you and have to keep reheating it. Even though they are slightly more expensive than other brands, I have found Thermacare[3] to be the best brand for the amount of skin surface they cover, for good adhesion, and staying warm the longest. They are usually available at Boots or online.

•You can apply creams such as Deep Heat or Deep Freeze to the affected muscles, which may give some short term pain relief. Studies have shown that these are not hugely effective, and I only use them as a convenient, short solution.

•If you prefer not to use a microwave, you can get gel packs which activate the heat when they have been submerged in hot water and a disk is then pressed. I saw some on sale and tried one out that would fit nicely around the neck and shoulders. These can be found on Amazon also.

3. www.thermacare.com

In the States, I paid for physiotherapy and was treated with more thorough sessions of hydrotherapy using very warm water, massage jets, and various weights to exercise with. One therapist also used to *'tape'* my upper back muscles to try and keep them from slouching and going into pain and spasm, and I found this helpful. She would also add in *'seeds'* which I believe were designed to press on certain acupressure points. These would stay attached to me for up to a week and did indeed help the upper back spasms.

You may be offered some of these treatments on the NHS and I say try anything! If it doesn't work for you however, don't think that a private alternative therapist offering a treatment under the same name will not work for you – approaches and methods in treatments vary greatly among practitioners and just need to be tried out, if you can afford it. I have had osteopaths and chiropractors treat me with infrared lamps, massage, the seeds I mentioned above, and homeopathic remedies... they all have different training and experience.

TENS MACHINE

Transcutaneous electrical nerve stimulation (TENS) is a method of pain relief involving the use of a mild electrical current, and is employed by physiotherapists if they think it necessary, and very often by midwives for women during the pains of labour. (It is mainly a therapeutic tool you can use by yourself, so could be in the *'practical management at home'* chapter, but it is widely recognised and used by the western medical establishment.)

I have had tens machines for years which involve a small electrical device like an iPod, that can fit in your pocket or clip onto a belt/jeans, with wires that lead to sticky pads called electrodes. You place the pads directly onto the skin on the area of pain (generally suitable for any back pain and best placed on the soft muscular areas rather than bones) and then turn on the current to your desired strength and pulse setting, which sends small electrical impulses to the area. Mine operates for 30 minutes before switch off, and then I usually turn it on again if needed. Depending on how sensitive my pain levels are, I can adjust the intensity at anytime. The pads last quite a while if they are looked after, but replacements are not too expensive and available from most good chemists. My original device only cost £15 and has served me very well, as well as during pregnancy and labour.

The electrical impulses can reduce the pain signals going to the spinal cord and brain, helping to relieve pain and relax muscles. It is thought they also stimulate the production of endorphins, which are the body's natural painkillers. If anything, I find that while the TENS machine is on, I can focus better on whatever activity I am trying to do, and also be completely mobile or sitting still. The wires can sometimes be a nuisance, or if I don't have any pockets or belt (when wearing a dress for instance). I know that wireless devices are now on the market – where you simply attach a whole sticky pad to the area of pain, and the controls are in the centre of the pad. I highly recommend this device to anyone with chronic back pain. A physiotherapist may be able to loan you a TENS machine for a trial period if they think it could help.

CHAPTER 3:

Exercise - Movement as Medicine

The majority of people reading this book are probably in pain most of the time, and/or almost constantly fatigued. (If you have ME or CFS, please see my footnotes as this is a different condition and may not respond well to the type of treatment approach I suggest for fibromyalgia and back pain[4]). The thought of exercise may cause you to hide under the duvet. But it is the one of ***the most important keys to managing pain***, as well as improving mental health and avoiding or managing episodes of depression which so often accompanies chronic pain. Exercise is also one of the first modes of treatment encouraged by fibromyalgia specialists, in order to reduce pain, improve fitness, cope with stress, and improve sleep.

---

4. In Myalgic encephalomyelitis or ME (As described in Canadian Consensus Document 2011 on ME/CFS), exercise and activity cause Post Exertional Malaise (PEM), a predominant symptom and diagnostic feature that is not present in other chronic illnesses.
PEM causes an increase in symptoms and exaggerated depletion in energy, after physical or mental exertion, either immediately or over the following days. This may present itself in different forms, from not being able to maintain normal levels of activity, all the way through to a total collapse and shut down of the body, both physically and cognitively. PEM may last hours, days, weeks or months.
Current research shows several possible reasons for PEM, including abnormalities in mitochondrial functions and increases in oxidative stress.
ME sufferers need to be aware that increases in activity must be approached carefully and slowly to avoid further debilitation. There is significant proof that pushing an ME sufferer to levels of activity that the body cannot cope with can cause permanent disability.
(Please note, due to current umbrella definitions of CFS (Chronic Fatigue Syndrome) or CFS/ME, some patients may not experience PEM as in classic ME. Chronic Fatigue, caused by other factors or conditions, may be helped by activity.) For further reading on this topic, see the bibliography.

I recommend reading Chapter 5 of 'The Fibromyalgia Handbook'[5] - Exercise Daily for Mobility and Energy. In there is included this diagram showing the cycle of activity:

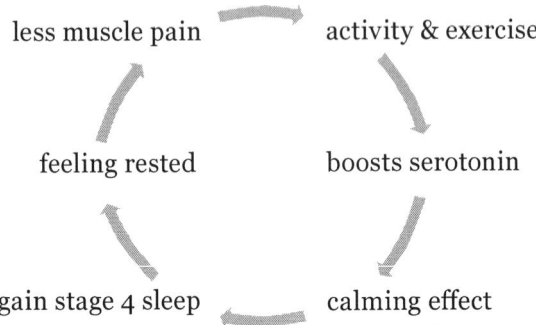

To start with, a new exercise regime might hurt. So whatever it is you chose to do, start safely and gently, but as long as it is suitable for your condition, don't give up... it might be swimming, walking, gentle dancing, yoga, Pilates, or cycling. Everyone is different and you will have to find what works for you the best. Have a strong mindset to give it a good go, with painkillers when necessary. When I was recovering from spinal surgery, there was no way I could have carried out my physiotherapy exercises without painkillers – but that is where you can use medication to enable you to do the exercise that will ultimately help you heal. Apart from receiving advice and knowing from personal experience that my body needs to move regularly, whenever I have prayed for guidance in managing this condition, I hear the words '*Exercise is Key*' over and over again.

I still experiment with different exercise programs or classes, if anything to keep it varied. The important point to remember is that movement is medicine, and even if for a minimum of 20 minutes each time, choose something suitable everyday to keep moving.

Exercise actually releases endorphins – feel good neurochemicals in your body that help to kill physical pain but also improve your mood, and we all know how important that is in living with pain.

5. Harris H.McIlwain, M.D & Debra Fulghum Bruce, Ph.D. © 1996 The Fibromyalgia Handbook. Holt Paperbacks p.98

Some days I exercise just because I know I'm feeling a bit low and need a pick me up, and if you can do it with a group of people, that may help even more. Exercise directly triggers the release of endorphins in the brain – these naturally produced endorphins actually resemble opium and its derivatives, such as heroin and morphine. People who exercise regularly therefore get more pleasure out of life – whereas the definition of depression is the absence of pleasure. Stimulating this neurological/hormone process with exercise also kindles the immune system and other physiological processes essential to all round health.[6]

> "Exercise gives you endorphins. Endorphins make you happy. Happy people just don't kill their husbands. They just don't."
>
> Elle Woods, 'Legally Blonde'

Exercise not only boosts levels of endorphins, but slows down the manufacture of excess adrenaline in the body that is associated with feeling stressed. *'Not only does exercise act as nature's tranquillizer, helping to boost serotonin levels in the brain, but studies show exercise also triggers the release of epinephrine and norepinephrine, which are known to boost alertness. For those who feel stressed out frequently, exercise will help to desensitize your body to stress*[7]*'*. Too much stress can also lead to low levels of serotonin, so exercise can help to prevent the feelings of depression that can come after a period of high stress.

A recent study published on the WebMD site suggests that exercise improves memory and pain levels in women with fibromyalgia, and in that I would include people with chronic back pain. The findings explain why regular exercise decreases pain and tenderness and improves brain function. Fibromyalgia, chronic pain, sleep problems, etc. can all cause less efficient memory and the ability to concentrate. Participants in the study who had been asked to give up their medication and then partake in an exercise program felt better physically and mentally than those in the control group, who had not taken part in exercise.

---

6. Read more in chapter 10 'Prozac or Puma?' Dr David Servan-Schrieber 'Healing without Freud or Prozac' ©2003, 2004, 2005. Rodale International Publishing.
7. Harris H.McIlwain, M.D & Debra Fulghum Bruce, Ph.D. © 1996 The Fibromyalgia Handbook. Holt Paperbacks p.101

Their brain scans *'observed a decrease in brain activity in areas that process pain and memory. This means the brain was more efficient and used less energy during a mental task. (Exercise) may help free up brain resources involved in perceiving pain and improve its ability to hold on to new information*[8]*'*.

Exercise also aids restful sleep, a crucial factor needed in managing pain (see chapter 3).

Self Discipline is the most important tool you need to keep exercising in a regular and healthy way, even on days you don't feel like it. Which, let's face it, could be most of the time for those in chronic pain. Discipline is what needs to be done, even if you don't want to or feel like doing it. *"I don't have time"* is the grown-up version of *"the dog ate my homework."* (Source unknown)

"You have to do right to feel right".

Michael Dye, the Genesis Process.

There is a fine line between needing to move, and overdoing it, however, and only you will be able to work that out through understanding what is *'good'* pain or bad pain. When muscles that are not used to moving in a certain way start to exercise, they might complain, so there is a certain amount of discomfort to be tolerated until you are stronger. *"Strength doesn't come from what you can do. It comes from overcoming the things you once thought you couldn't".* (Source unknown)

In my experience, with fibromyalgia, these muscles seem to complain for much longer than a healthy person's would. That is where heat, ice, rest and painkillers are needed so that you can keep exercising, sensibly. If you take so many painkillers that they mask the pain and you go at it like an athlete – you will obviously pay for it when the effects have worn off! You will get to know your limits with a bit of practice.

---

8. Cari Nierenberg. 'Exercise May Improve Memory in Fibromyalgia Patients'. Study Shows Physical Activity Helps the Brain Work More Efficiently and Eases Pain. WebMD Health News. Reviewed by Michael W. Smith, MD www.webmd.com/fibromyalgia/news/20111117/exercise-may-improve-memory-in-fibromyalgia-patients?

Also, stretching muscles is essential, but can be quite uncomfortable – this is what I call 'good pain' when you can feel it being stretched out and lengthening, but not spasming. Some trainers advise that you should stretch before a workout – I have found that my muscles need to be warmed up before being stretched, so I do it either after a gentle warm up, and/or at the end. Alternatively exercising straight after a hot shower can help since the muscles have been warmed. If you think of a cold elastic band being stretched – it is brittle and can easily snap, however if it is warm it is much more flexible – muscles work in the same way.

I have included some rough sketches my favourite stretches for back pain, and for me – they are ESSENTIAL and have just become part of my daily movement – vocabulary. Other more cardiovascular forms of exercise are to be performed on top of these and need a little more time set aside to do. There are many other types of stretches that you can be taught by a physiotherapist, or a Pilates or yoga teacher, and please do get the advice of professionals who can watch you perform, to make sure you do them correctly.

SIMPLE BACK STRETCHES

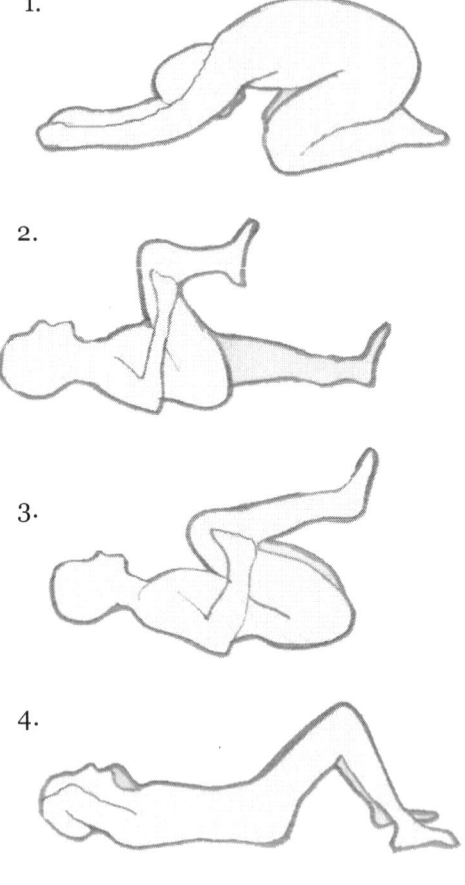

1. CHILD POSE
Sit on the floor with your knees bent, and your buttocks on your heels. Walk your hands out in front of you, lowering your torso so your belly is resting on your thighs. Extend your arms as much as possible for a lower back stretch*

2. SINGLE KNEE HUG
Lie flat and simply hug each knee towards the chest, one at a time, holding for up to 30 seconds for a lower back stretch.

3. DOUBLE KNEE HUG
If the pain isn't too great, also repeat the knee hug with both legs.

4. PELVIC TILT
Lie on your back with knees bent. "Brace" your stomach - tighten your muscles by pulling in and imagining your belly button moving toward your spine. Hold for about 6 seconds while breathing smoothly.

Repeat 8 to 12 times.

*To stretch each side whilst in child pose, also keep the right hand where it is and lift your left hand and place it to the right of your right pinky. Lower your head and just breathe. Repeat on the other side.

Note Those with neck injuries should keep the head in line with the torso, not dropping it forward or back. Pregnant women and those with back injuries should only perform Cow Pose, bringing the spine back to neutral between poses - do not let the belly drop between repetitions, as this can strain the lower back.

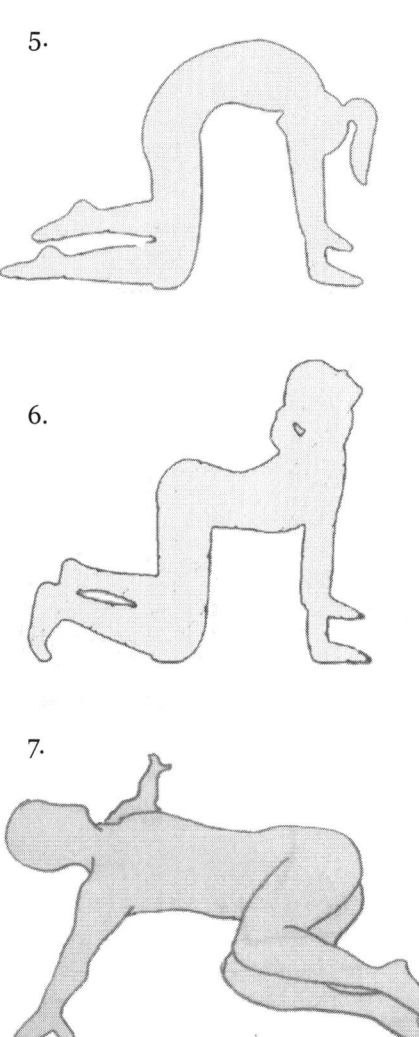

5. CAT TO COW STRETCH**

Start on your hands and knees with your wrists directly under your shoulder, and your knees directly under your hips, hips-width apart. Centre your head in a neutral position and soften your gaze downward. Begin by moving into Cat Pose. As you exhale, draw your belly to your spine and round your back toward the ceiling. Release the crown of your head toward the floor, but don't force your chin to your chest.

6. MOVE INTO COW POSE.

Inhale as you drop your belly towards the mat. Lift your chin and chest, and gaze up toward the ceiling. Broaden across your shoulder blades and draw your shoulder away from your ears. Exhale as you return to Cat Pose. Repeat 5-20 times.

7. SPINAL TWIST

While on your back, hug your knees to your chest. Whilst engaging your abs and keeping your back supported, gently bring your knees down to your right side. Now, gently look left. Draw the knees up back to centre, using the abs to do this. Repeat on your other side.

8.

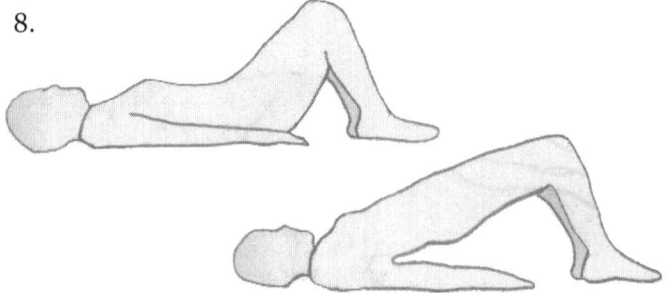

8. PELVIC BRIDGE WITH NEUTRAL SPINE.

Lie with your knees bent and your feet planted in the ground. Inhale into the back of your ribs, and then exhale as you lift your pelvis into the air. Inhale, fold at the hip sockets to lower the ribcage and tail-bone gradually (bone by bone) to the floor. Exhale as you lift your pelvis. Imagine you are sending your knees over your toes. Exhale as you lift your pelvis and inhale as you lower your tail-bone and ribcage sequentially to the ground.

9.

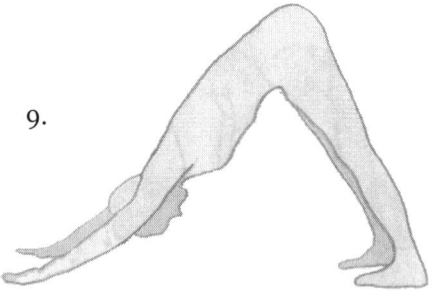

9. DOWN DOG

Beginning on your hands and knees, align wrists directly under shoulders and knees directly under hips. Point middle fingers towards top edge of mat, and spread fingers wide. Relax your upper back. Press firmly through your hands and exhale as you tuck your toes and lift your pelvis up to the ceiling. Draw your sit bones to the wall behind you. Straighten legs as much as possible without locking the knees. Press the floor away as you continue to lift through the pelvis, lengthening your spine. Align your ears with your upper arms and relax your head, not letting it dangle. Release gently to lower back down to hands and knees.

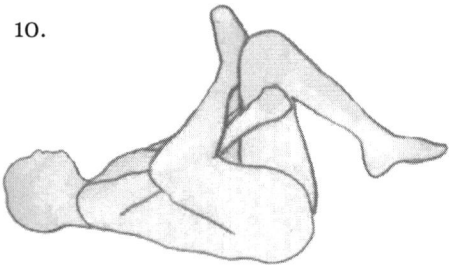

10. HIP AND BUTTOCK STRETCH
Lie on your back with feet off the floor and cross right ankle over left knee. Grasp the back of left thigh and gently pull legs towards the chest, stretching the right hip and buttock. Take 3 deep breathes, change sides and repeat.

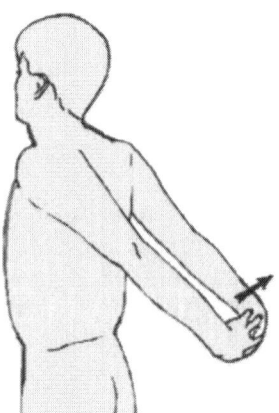

11. CHEST STRETCH
Standing with feet shoulder width apart, pull arms behind your chest, pressing shoulder blades together and feeling a stretch across the pectoral muscles (collar bone and front chest). Hold it there and breathe for a few seconds before releasing.

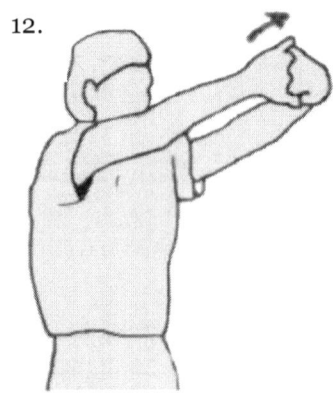

12. CHEST STRETCH 2
Standing upright with hands extended in front of your chest. Interlace fingers and push them away from your chest, until you feel a stretch in your upper back. Hold it there and breathe for a few seconds before releasing.

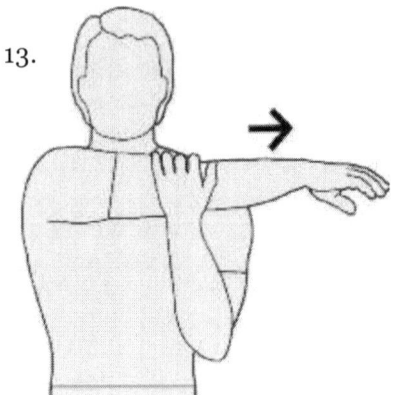

13. SHOULDER AND UPPER ARM STRETCH
Put one arm, straightened, in front of you and cross over directly under your chin. With the other hand, gently push the arm closer to your body.

Repeat on the other side.

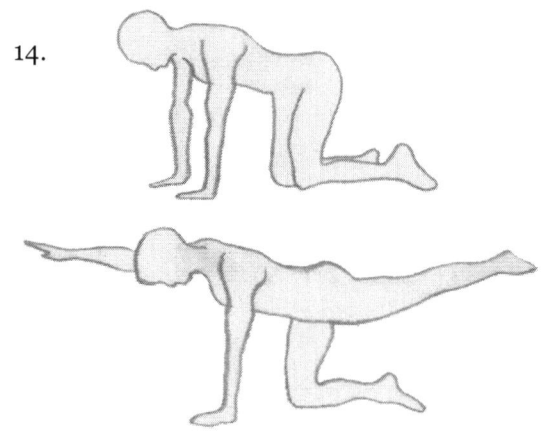

14. KNEELING ARM AND LEG REACH

Kneel on all fours with arms directly under shoulders, knees under hips, and spine neutral. Keeping the abs pulled in and torso steady, reach one arm forward and the alternative leg back, keeping fingers and toes on ground. Lift the extending leg and arm into a straight line, remaining stable through the core. Hold for a few seconds then lower and repeat on the other side.

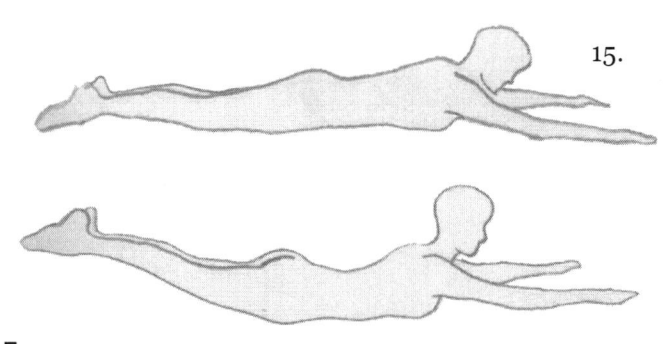

15.

This move is to strengthen the lower back, and prepares you for a Pilates 'Swimming' exercise, which should not be done when the back is weak/in a flare up. Lie on stomach with legs and arms extended. Engage abs. Gently lift arms and legs off the floor, and hover nose about mat (do not over extend the neck). Hold, or move into swimming action (see Pilates teacher for this), and release. *Note that over extension of the spine could be detrimental to some people with back pain.*

images here edited from 2createabody.com and womensheart.com

WALKING

I cannot stress enough that this has been one of the most important tools in my daily fight against back pain. But my ability to use it varies from day to day, and unfortunately since having spinal surgery my walking ability has reduced instead of increased, but I still do it. The body has to move - the spine definitely has to move, in order to stay healthy. If I have to sit for any length of time, I will take regular breaks to walk around, wiggle, stretch, etc. If I feel well enough to walk to the local shop rather than driving that day, I will walk, and take a shopping trolley or something with wheels to carry any slightly heavy bags.

If your condition allows you to walk – walk as much as you can without causing a lot more pain, everyday. It might be 5-10 minutes, it might be 40 minutes, but do what you can. If it causes significant pain whilst walking, then stop. If you are sore afterwards, note how long it takes you to recover. If you feel fine the next day, you can repeat it, or increase it slightly. If it takes longer than 1 day to recover, perhaps reduce the distance next time and play around with how much walking will make you feel better rather than worse.

FOOTWEAR

The type of footwear you walk in is just as important as how long you walk for. Wear good quality walking shoes or running trainers, which have more shock-absorbency than regular leather shoes. Have your feet assessed for the type of arch you naturally have and how you can avoid more back, hip, leg or foot pain by wearing the right kind of insole. You can often get a free assessment in a chiropody approved footwear store that sells or provides custom-made insoles. Or ask your GP or pain clinic if an NHS assessment for insoles is possible.

I have a high arch, and therefore must have footwear with good arch support or wear an insole that was made for me. Therefore flat pretty shoes from general high street shops, or high heels, are out of the question for me. I resigned myself long ago to only buying decent footwear with arch support and shock absorbent soles in the likes of brands such as Hotter, Clarks, Reiker, and Joseph Seibel, Fly.... They aren't cheap, but your health is worth it. For a more trainer-type shoe or plimsoll, which I find ***incredibly*** comfortable, I wear Sketchers, and own about 5 different pairs! They have increased their range of styles, from funky to more conventional 'sensible' designs, so can suit all ages.

YOGA

If you, like me, are a Christian, or it interests/concerns you, please also see my section on *'Considering the Spiritual Implications of alternative therapies'*.

Yoga practices has it's roots as far back as 4000 BC in India, but is practised today worldwide. It is a holistic practice, intended to effect the physical, mental and spiritual sides of a person. There are five different types of yoga: raja, jnana, karma, bakti and hatha. Hatha yoga is the most popular form practiced in the west, and involves the use of exercises and positions; The other forms of yoga have more to do with matters of the mind, intellect and morality. Correct breathing is an important element of yoga – it is believed that the body's life essence, or *'prana'*, is in the breath. Controlled breathing should therefore promote a healthier state physically, mentally and emotionally. This is one reason why it is good to attend a class where there is a well trained yoga teacher who can observe and correct the way you perform the exercises and breathing.

Some Yoga routines or practicing a series of stretching poses can be very helpful if you experience sore muscles on a regular basis. Stretching helps to lubricate the joints, and send nutrients and oxygen to the muscles, as well as helping to reduce stress and potentially the need for as many medications.

I have gone to many classes on/off over the years – because sometimes it would just hurt too much for days afterwards, or there were exercises I didn't feel were appropriate for my particular back pain, and so I would not want to return. Also if the classes were too *'spiritually'* orientated that would put me off, but there are classes that are led as a purely physical exercise class. The body can move and pose in certain ways to benefit core and outer health and appearance; it doesn't have to be made into a spiritual exercise, and saying that, it is possible to utilise some of the helpful poses from yoga in your own daily stretching, without taking part in an actual yoga group/

class (The examples of illustrated back exercises on previous pages incorporate stretches I learned from yoga and Pilates). Bear in mind that reaching a calm and positive state of mind through breathing and poses, is always going to help manage pain or tension.

There are *so many* poses in yoga and most that can be customized to suit your body. The expertise and sensitivity of a good teacher is essential, and so if you choose to try yoga, you might need to shop around. If budget permits, many teachers offer one-to-one sessions.

YouTube is also an excellent resource for trying yoga at home. That way if something really hurts, you can leave it out or customize the movement without being self-conscious. I do find it much more helpful and beneficial to practice along with gentle music, though, so if the video does not have music on it, play some in the background.

When I do go through phases of trying to do more regular, small bouts of stretches I have picked up from yoga/Pilates, I am amazed how much better my back can feel for a day or two afterwards, as well as feeling less fatigued. In particular, I find the child pose, down dog, and mountain pose very helpful for me and perform them most days.

PILATES

'If practiced regularly, Pilates improves flexibility, builds strength and endurance. It emphasizes proper alignment, breathing, and developing a strong core. This core, referring to the muscles of the abdomen, low back, and hips, is often called the "powerhouse" - key to a person's stability'.

Pilates is a physical fitness system developed by Joseph Pilates in the early 20th century, as a way of overcoming his own ailments and illnesses as a child. In short, it is training in the art of controlled movements during a workout. Pilates emphasizes core strength and stability, which is so important for those susceptible to back pain. Pilates teacher Sarah Lloyd Clary explains:

"Recent developments in scanning technology have confirmed what Joseph Pilates knew, that by focusing on breathing and the mechanics of the body you can help to strengthen your body from the inside out and return your body to a place of balance. This makes Pilates an excellent choice for participants looking to rehabilitate after injury or to manage joint pain, especially lower back pain.

Pilates focuses on the body as a whole and aims to build good postural alignment. We begin by bringing our attention to the core muscles of body (The Pelvic Floor, the Diaphragm, the Transverse abdominis and the multifidus in the spine) these intrinsic muscles are important in reducing lower back pain as they stabilise the trunk and pelvis and protect the vertebrae in your lumbar spine. Then by focusing on the Pilates breathing techniques you release stiffness in the ribcage, the act of focusing totally on breath can be relaxing and calming[9]".

Joint health, flexibility and posture are all important factors too, and to ensure you are doing the exercises precisely, a teacher who can observe and correct you is much safer than trying at home with a DVD or YouTube to begin with. Chronic pain itself can cause postural changes that need the correction of a professional; "The period of immobility causes some muscles to weaken and others to become over-tight, creating even more imbalance over time than the original injury or stress. A good teacher will be able to observe a client as they move and recognise their posture type and the areas of the body that are tight or weak. They will give movements to the client that are specific to their needs and are achievable and safe, layering on technique and challenge as the client is ready".

There is so much to discover in Pilates, I highly recommend you attend a class by a well-trained practitioner who understands back problems and fibromyalgia, if possible. Again, over the years I have attended a range of classes – some which hurt and I never went back! Others that I practiced religiously twice a

9. Sarah Lloyd-Clary, SLC Pilates Teacher in Bath UK.
www.facebook.com/pg/SLC-Pilates

week because I believed they helped so much – before and after major spinal surgery.

Some teachers are general gym instructors who have done a short course in Pilates, and may not offer classes suitable for those with injuries. If you can, check what training they have had. Stott trained Pilates teachers are an excellent choice, or those who work in osteopathy or physiotherapy centres as well.

There are still some exercises I leave out because I find them too painful for my back or neck, but that isn't to say you won't be able to do them. Do find a sympathetic but well educated Pilates coach.

TAI CHI & CHI GONG

I have not had much experience of these practices, partly because of the lack of availability in my area, and not feeling competent enough at first to do it by myself with a DVD or YouTube. However a few alternative health care professionals have suggested it would be good for me. It is slow, very precise, and gentle, so would suit any level of ability.

Both Tai Chi and Chi Gong are ancient Chinese healing practices which combine meditation, dance, movement, and breathing techniques. Studies show they can improve energy, lessen fatigue, and ease pain. I encourage you to try them out if you think it would suit you. I have read many positive testimonials from those who practice them. This form of movement can suit fibromyalgia sufferers who find exercise painful. Both Tai Chi and Chi Gong involve slowly moving the body in a full range of motion and can also help reduce stress levels. However it is hard to learn from a book or DVD, and you should attend a class for one to one instruction. Classes will usually begin with a period of meditative stillness before progressing through very specific movements led by the hands and feet.

The ultimate goal of Tai Chi is to bring the principles of yin and yang into natural harmony, and it is thought to have originated with the meditation of a Taoist monk, and the aim of practising is to surrender to the natural flow of the universe and become one with it.[10] You may want to look into the spiritual background of it before practicing; if you are concerned about that aspect – see my chapter on *Considering the Spiritual in Alternative Therapies*.

SWIMMING

If one more person tells me that "swimming is the best form of exercise for back pain", I might clobber them! In the early days of my search for relief, I spent a lot of time splashing around in the pool, with very bad form and technique, so that I actually made the pain worse. In particular my neck and shoulders suffered more for many days afterwards and I would be left with big muscle knots that could only be relieved by deep massage, muscle relaxants, heat, etc..

Probably swimming is one of the best forms of exercise – if done properly. So I am trying to learn to swim with good posture, and the ability to keep my neck in line with my spine (head in water) without swallowing and snorting a pint for every 2 strokes! Especially since I am currently in my second pregnancy, gentle swimming – particularly on my back – is necessary to manage pain. And I must say I never feel like going! I could almost say I hate the thought of it – getting undressed and dressed, lowering into cold water for exercise I don't particularly enjoy. But as long as I do it properly and don't use my neck and shoulders too much, I nearly always feel better for the rest of the day and the day after, so it is worth it. (Yet so far, if I do more than a few lengths of breast stroke, my neck and shoulders go into spasm for days afterwards).

The buoyancy of water means that body weight is supported, which brings some relief, and exercising in water is often safer on the joints. I have found swimming in calm salt water easier, because it causes you to float more - but we can't all access the likes of Olu Deniz blue lagoon in Turkey on a regular basis!

Exercising in warm water is far easier and more pain-relieving than in cold water, so pick a day that the swimming pool might raise the temperature (for when senior citizens or babies swim) or attend a hydrotherapy pool. Hydrotherapy pools open to public use or in hospital physiotherapy departments, have been one of the best resources for me in my quest for healing. There is nothing like gentle movement in warm water for sore muscles. Do see if this is something a GP can refer you for, or contact a pool directly to see if you can self-refer. When pregnant, Aqua Natal in the Royal United Hospital pool (Bath, UK) got me through - It

---

10. Geddes & Grosset. Guide to Natural Healing. © 2005 Tai Chi Ch'uan, p. 145

was the one day a week I always had significantly less pain. And post-spinal surgery, this was the best form of exercise for my recovery.

THE GYM

This is a tricky one to discuss in a book. Depending on your particular disability, you will need to find machinery that you can exercise on with minimal discomfort, but that increases your muscle strength and mobility. All gyms offer an induction and the trainer should be able to advise you accordingly, but you may need to invest in a few personal training sessions as well, being sure that the trainer has a good understanding of fibromyalgia and chronic pain.

If you have been through a pain clinic program, they should have taught you there about what would be good for you and you will have tried out some of the equipment in the physiotherapy department. For me, any high impact exercise, like the running machine, worsens my back pain during and after exercise. The rowing machine is also another one I stay away from because of back problems. But appropriate strength training with light weights is important to try and build muscle strength, although I often experience muscle spasms in my shoulders when lifting weights and so take it very gently, and stop when my muscles start 'pinching' rather than contracting.

Regular (at least twice weekly) use of the cross trainer for mobility in my back and also getting into the cardiovascular realm of exercise, is a must for me.

The cross trainer causes the upper and lower body to move, without high impact. It is important to keep your core muscles switched on and to have good upright posture when cross training, and make sure the knees don't turn inwards. I also prefer to keep my heels flat on the platform. During times when I have not been to the gym to use the cross trainer, my back pain has definitely become more unmanageable. Some days I am so sore in either my back or hips that I can only manage up to 5 minutes, but that is better than nothing. I take pain killers if necessary in order to do this bit of exercise which I know will benefit me later. On a good day I can do 15 minutes, but if you can do more without suffering a great deal in the following days, then great! Before I had back surgery, ironically, I could go for longer, but now my hips prevent me.

There are many other cardiovascular and weight training machines to be found in a regular gym, but do get personalised advice appropriate for your condition, and supervision by a physiotherapist or personal trainer when starting out a new exercise.

CYCLING

These days I don't do a lot of this, due to my hip problems, but I do find short cycle rides in fine weather quite therapeutic, and I used to go for 30 minute rides in the early days of having back pain. As long as I had good posture, I always used to find cycling would not exacerbate it, and would release endorphins. That's why I now have a Dutch lady's bike that I can sit up straight on, rather than bent over handle bars. Gel seat covers are awesome! And make sure the seat is the correct height for you – the leg should not be over-extended when the pedal is down. Have a physiotherapist or trained personnel in a bike shop show you the best height for you. Spinning classes are widely available at most gyms – again you need to try this for yourself to see if it would help or exacerbate your pain levels.

There are obviously other forms of exercise that may help you, but I have only discussed those that I use. Any form of high impact exercise – i.e. running or jumping, aerobics and Zumba, etc., are not suitable for my type of spine problem and may not suit you either. Try it out and listen to your body.

Do also consider if some forms of dancing might suit you, as this is certainly good for lifting the spirits. I did occasionally go to Ceroc – a dance movement in the UK that combines a mixture of ballroom and modern jive, but I can only go with painkillers, caffeine, and then I only dance to the slower songs and not the jumpy ones. Now with me having hip pain, it does usually cause flare up, yet it actually doesn't always make the back pain worse, as long as I avoid back-bends or limboing! The dance class gets me out, I adore watching others dance whilst I take rests; I have made wonderful friends through the classes, and even met my husband!

If you are busy with something you enjoy, then the pain can be displaced to have less prominence in your thoughts and feelings.

CHAPTER 4:

Pain Clinics

If you have been in chronic pain for some time and go to the GP for help, then they may refer you to a pain management program at the local hospital, called the Pain Clinic. I would recommend taking this opportunity if you are able; it is usually for a period of 6-8 weeks, once a week. You can expect to join a group of other patients with various chronic pain problems, and together you will explore ways of coping, exercising, some elements of CBT (Cognitive Behavioural Therapy) etc.. Becoming aware of how our particular thoughts and feelings affect our activity and pain levels, and how to manage the interactive relationship between these four factors, is a major and helpful part of the course.

Pain affects all areas of our lives, the things we do, the things we think, and the things we feel. However, our activities, thoughts and feelings also affect the level of pain we experience. The aim of the pain clinic program is to teach us to have control over these three areas so that pain can be managed by us, the sufferer, rather than IT controlling us.

Unlike acute pain, which is like a warning that we have damaged our tissues and need to do something to allow healing to take place, chronic pain is long-lasting and there is not always evidence that tissue damage is occurring - it is useless pain because it is not telling us anything important. In chronic pain, doing things that are good for us that might hurt, does not always equal harm.

The pain clinic team will usually consist of a group of trained professionals such as a physiotherapist, clinical psychologist, occupational therapist, anaesthetist, and a nurse. They are ready to help you understand, accept and manage your illness, pain and fatigue, and learn to have a better quality of life. You can learn that although you can't do as much as 'normal' people, a balance can be achieved between doing those things that you have to and making time for things you want to do. People who are also fatigued and in pain will also tend to avoid activities which actually could be helpful, done in moderation. The pain clinic team will try and help people out of a 'rut' if they are stuck in a cycle of avoidance behaviours.

Another part of the day at the pain clinic was a relaxation session, whereby we were taught to try and relax every part of our body and enter into a more calm and pain-free state. Teaching correct diaphragmatic breathing is a big part of this; taking deep slow breaths can immediately stimulate the parasympathetic nervous system and help to give a bit of a physiological 'break'.

To take a deep diaphragmatic breath, imagine your lungs filling with air as you breath in through your nose. The stomach should come out a little bit if the diaphragm is being used correctly. When the lungs are completely full, gently exhale fully and completely. In a group relation session we might be encouraged to imagine each intake of oxygen nourishing the body and each exhalation ridding the body of waste products, and pain and stress. It is a good idea to have an experienced person check you are doing this properly (Alexander therapists, yoga or Pilates teaches, etc. may also be able to help) and then use it as a daily tool for relaxation.

In 1965, two scientists, Ronald Melzack and Patrick Wall, developed something called the Pain Gate Theory. Gates can be opened or closed, and in the case of lower back pain, for example, the gate concerned is in the nerves of the spinal cord in the lower back. Factors which open the pain gate can be depression, rest, or overdoing things.

The brain can influence how open or shut the pain gates are; if we are depressed, messages come down from the brain and make the gate nerves more excitable - causing more pain transmission. During rest, messages normally coming in from muscles and joints are reduced, so more pain messages can be delivered. If we overdo things, strong pain messages going into the spinal cord lower our threshold - exciting the pain gate nerves to allow more pain messages to be transmitted to the brain. *'By overdoing things we are changing the chemistry of our nerves to make them transmit pain more easily, which makes us more disabled without any damage occurring. By pacing, the nerves can be retrained to respond less dramatically to impulses coming in*[11].

By learning to pace activities, we can avoid overdoing things, so that the pain gates never get a huge blast of sensations which make the nerves excitable so easily.

So we can do something ourselves about pain gates in order to cause them to close. Not only pacing, but distraction is a great tool that I use every day to close my pain gates - if you are busy with something you enjoy, then the pain can be displaced to have less prominence in our thoughts and feelings. This is the reason I try to engross myself in hobbies such as arts and crafts. Regular appropriate exercise can dampen the excitability of nerves and make pain transmission less effective.

Some medications work by altering the amount of messages transmitted in the pain gates/brain, and the different types might be described in much more detail by an anaesthetist at the pain clinic.

I did my first pain management course in Exeter and found the team especially helpful, teaching me skills I have used ever since. I was fortunate in later years to move to Bath, where they have the National Hospital for Rheumatic Diseases – The Mineral Hospital, or "Min". The professional health care team there understood the nature of chronic pain, and fibromyalgia, really well, and I found them to be supportive. They offered me hydrotherapy sessions, cortisol injections, further physiotherapy (assessing my exercises); tried out various medications, and finally I had a caudal epidural injection in my spine. The injections did not work for me and were incredibly painful, but they do work for some people.

Attending a pain clinic is a great way of learning to pace our activity in order to manage pain better, and the professionals there will give you individualized advice.

---

11. The Pain Gate. Handout from the Royal Devon & Exeter Healthcare NHS Trust

SECTION II

Alternative Therapies

I will now move on to talk about what are generally considered in the western world to be *'alternative'* and complementary treatments, although some are now incorporated and adopted into the treatment approach taken by the more conventional practitioners in western medicine (e.g. physiotherapists, even some GPs).

The main issue that some people have with considering whether to use an alternative therapy is that most therapies have little compelling scientific evidence to support their effectiveness, or ambiguous evidence, based on flawed studies. Often, the only evidence is a group of testimonials – personal and thus non-subjective accounts of how a therapy has helped or cured the individual. Nevertheless, therapies used for centuries in other cultures would surely not have gained acceptance if they were not effective?

If you try a new therapy, a *'proposed cure'*. or even a new pharmaceutical medication, bear in mind the power of the placebo effect (the belief that it will work).

CHAPTER 5:

Physical Manipulation Therapies

Chiropractic, Osteopathy and Osteomyology are the main *'manipulation therapies'* whereby the practitioner will assess the patient's spine and posture, and try to move the bones around or encourage certain muscles to relax in order to relieve pain.

I won't go into too much detail about these treatments because each practitioner is different, and I had a different outcome depending on who I saw, as well as just what my pain levels were doing at the time! Do be aware that these practitioners are often keen to see you regularly, and may give you a *'diagnosis'* of misaligned hips, or one leg shorter than the other, for example, to make you feel like they know exactly what is wrong with you. They want you to return for treatment because of course that is how they make their money. Although some will be generally honest and say if they don't think you need to be seen for a while.

Having misaligned hips is actually very common in people with back or hip pain – when we are in pain we might overcompensate and take more weight on one side when walking, for example, and this *'puts'* things out of line. It is therefore usually beneficial to get this treated by physical manipulation, and then to strengthen the muscles and correct postural habits so that you can stay in the right alignment. Seeing such a therapist should be used as part of a management program – to set things right and be educated about your body, but also to keep up the correct exercises.

CHIROPRACTIC

Chiropractic is concerned with the diagnosis and treatment of unverified mechanical disorders of the musculoskeletal system, especially the spine, with the belief that such disorders can affect health via the nervous system. It usually involves manual therapy, manipulating the spine or other joints and soft tissues. I visited many different chiropractors in the early years of my back pain - both in the UK and USA, and their techniques do vary. Some have a very mechanical, biological approach to treatment, and a few can be more spiritual / existentialist in their approach. Some chiropractors "employ conventional treatments including physical therapy such as exercise, stretching, massage, ice packs, electrical muscle stimulation, therapeutic ultrasound, and moist heat.[12] Some also use alternative techniques, including nutritional supplements, acupuncture, homeopathy, herbal remedies, and biofeedback[13]".

Generally after chiropractic treatment, depending on how much manipulation was done and with what force, I would tend to be sore for a few days afterward – it was a different pain to what I went in for, however. Ice and rest and painkillers would generally help me recover, and sometimes I noticed reduced chronic back pain afterwards for a few days or even a week, but it never seemed to last, so I would return for another recommended treatment, spending more money.

OSTEOPATHY

The NHS website describes Osteopathy as *'a way of detecting, treating and preventing health problems by moving, stretching and massaging a person's muscles and joints. Osteopathy is based on the principle that the well-being of an individual depends on their bones, muscles, ligaments and connective tissue functioning smoothly together[14]'.*

---

12. Kaptchuk TJ, Eisenberg DM (November 1998). "Chiropractic: origins, controversies, and contributions". Arch. Intern. Med. 158 (20): 2215–24. PMID 9818801
13. Martin SC (October 1993). "Chiropractic and the social context of medical technology, 1895-1925". Technol Cult. 34 (4): 808–34. JSTOR 3106416. PMID 11623404
14. www.nhs.uk/conditions/osteopathy/pages/introduction.aspx

Osteopaths use physical manipulation, stretching and massage, in order to increase mobility, relieve tight muscles and enhance blood flow to tissues so that the body can heal itself. I mostly had positive experiences from visiting osteopaths, and didn't experience so much *'soreness'* and the need to recover afterwards, as compared with my experience with chiropractic treatments. I found it especially helpful if I was experiencing muscle spasms in my upper back, neck and shoulders, and sometimes the only treatment that would release the spasm. After back surgery I did not attend any manipulation treatments for fear that they might 'undo' any fixing of the spine. However I am considering attending again, given the funds to do so. A lot of people with back pain find they need to attend a few sessions during an acute attack of pain, and then go less regularly for *'maintenance'*.

OSTEOMYOLOGY

Osteomyologists are members of a relatively new group of 'manipulation therapy' practitioners who are trained in a variety of techniques so that they can customise treatment according to the patient's condition and symptoms. The osteomyologist I visited regularly, (and found the treatment to be very helpful) was actually a trained chiropractor who had trained in other areas as well. Following the Chiropractic Act 1994, and the Osteopaths Act 1993, she did not welcome the new registration and governing requirements needed to protect her title of chiropractor; so many osteomyologists use these techniques but just can't describe themselves as Osteopaths or Chiropractors. She would also recommend certain exercises and give postural advice, as well as suggest a homeopathic or herbal remedy that might help. Unfortunately I live too far away to attend treatment with her now, but also, as with many of these therapies, I needed it every few weeks where possible, and it was costly.

CRANIAL OSTEOPATHY

Cranial osteopathy is not too different from osteopathy, but is a subtle and refined approach following the same principles, and simply refers to the fact that it includes the gentle manipulation of the bones of the skull. Practitioners use their sense of touch to feel tensions or poor tissue quality in the anatomy of the whole body, and try to release those areas and allow them to heal, using gentle manipulation of the bones in the head. It can feel like not much is happening during the treatment, apart from a sense of relaxation, but just because you can't feel or see the subtle changes happening in the bones and flow of the spinal fluid, it doesn't mean cranial osteopathy doesn't work.

I believe these physical manipulation treatments are worth a try, if you can afford it, and as long as the practitioner is highly trained and regulated.

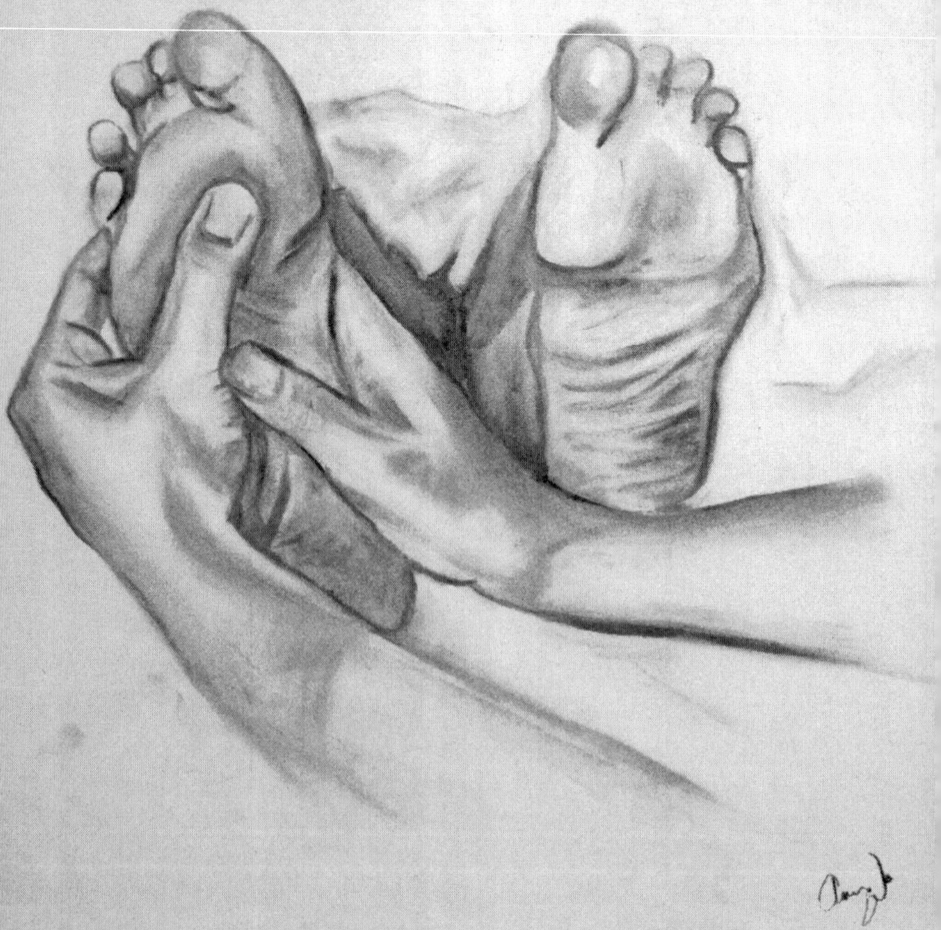

CHAPTER 6:

Massage

I have to say I would not manage pain or cope with it without receiving massage therapy, along with appropriate exercise. There are so many different types of massage – Swedish, hot stone, aromatherapy, sports, deep tissue, Indian head.... the list goes on, so do experiment with a style that suits your body and pain levels, or tolerance of touch. For me, most types of massage are very pleasant to receive, but Swedish or deep tissue massage has proved the most effective in releasing tight muscles and therefore pain, and the one I keep going back for.

Pain and stress can make muscles more tense, having built up excess lactic acid. Massage is one of the only ways to release this and is therefore, in my opinion, the most important treatment for back pain and other muscular pains and spasms. Other benefits of massage include:

improved mood

improved alertness

better sleep

reduction in the level of cortisol (the stress hormone)

helps reduce need for pain killers, muscle relaxants and sedatives

increased circulation

increased mobility

better digestion

relaxes the nervous system

reduces anxiety

releases endorphins.

Artwork, 'Massage' by Amy Jo Haskins (Samuel). Graphite & Charcoal. 2017 www.amyjo-arts.co.uk

Having listed all those benefits, why wouldn't you find an appropriate form of massage that helps your particular pain problem, and have regular treatments? The answer often lies in the cost of treatments, so shop around, or see if there is someone who may treat from their own home (bringing the cost down) on a regular basis. For me, it is so worth the cost because of all the benefits listed above, which makes for a happier and more productive days following the treatment.

For affordable massage, it is worth looking at your local college to see if students on beauty courses can treat you at very competitive prices. I have had many great massages and trialled some other treatments within these colleges, and only a couple of mediocre experiences.

To try and save the cost of regular massage and to be able to access it anytime, we invested in a highly technological Inada[15] massage chair, designed by the Japanese, and only available through their sales representatives. We chose the one that has attachments that also work the feet, lower legs, and arms as well as the rest of the body.

The chair works on the principles of traditional Japanese shiatsu/acupressure and is a huge chair that can be used in the convenience of your own home, where you control the types of massage and which part of the body you would like focused on. It has many different programs to suit your preferences, pressure, massage style. The bottom line is, most of it feels nice, it is relaxing, and great to use in the evenings. However, although if used regularly it is more effective at preventing or managing muscle pain, and can aid sleep, it doesn't seem to take away a chronic pain or upper back spasm quite like a real hands-on massage.

I have also bought quite a few hand held massage devices. If you ever visit the 'Back Show[16]' or any pain relief exhibition, you will see many new inventions all designed to change your life and remove pain, by treating yourself at home. I can't say I have been satisfied with any of them - but I'm always comparing it to how real massage helps me, and I'm sure home devices help some people.

15. www.inada.co.uk
16. www.thebackpainshow.co.uk

I even bought an 'acupen' which you can use on yourself to apply an electrical current to relevant acupressure points or trigger points on the body. It generally comes with a guide and you can download a map of the body with all the appropriate points. I was finding acupuncture treatments very beneficial, and so this was my attempt to save money on attending the treatments. I am unsure I spent enough time and commitment to give it a good go, to be honest. I tried, but to no avail. I think it is worth a shot, but better if a carer or family member can use it on you whilst you relax, and you do need to have time set aside to attend to the various points on your body.

You can also take time to self-massage your hands and feet, with a base carrier oil such as sweet almond oil, and perhaps a few drops of aromatherapy oil. This can help relax you and massage out any obvious 'knots' in the feet and hands. Bathing in a warm, Epsom salts bath beforehand would also help for muscle aches and pains.

REFLEXOLOGY

I have included this topic here because it can be classed as a type of massage; Reflexology merely uses a specific type of massage at a specific location on the body to treat symptoms and induce a state of health and relaxation. The body's energy is thought to flow along certain routes, connecting every organ and gland with an end point on the feet, hands, or another part of the body (including the ear). If a certain route is blocked, those end points can be tender, and the massaging of particular reflex points can help clear the blockage. The premise of this treatment is, when pain is experienced in one part of the body, it can be relieved by applying pressure elsewhere in the body.

Although I believe in some of the biological principles of reflexology, I have not received a treatment – mainly due to the cost of it, being a little wary of the spiritual background of the practice, and because I know full body massage is one of the best things for me, I saved my money for that.

In its 20th Century form, reflexology divided the body into ten vertical zones running from feet to head, and down each arm. Believing energy to flow through each zone, the energy must be balanced in order for the organs in that zone to function well. Imbalances in this energy field lead to waste material (such as uric acid and calcium crystals) building up in the reflex points. The reflex points for all parts of the body are located on the feet, so pressure is applied to break up these unhealthy accumulations, which allegedly restores health to the corresponding parts of the body.

Reflexology is also thought to increase blood flow to the corresponding body parts and thus eliminate toxins, so it doesn't necessarily have to be viewed as just an energy therapy based on traditional Chinese medicine. But some therapists interpret their work in terms of life energy manipulation, which Christians may want to be cautious of. This is another reason why I have not tried reflexology though I would not rule it out, depending on the practitioner's beliefs and approach.

I did have Thai foot massage, both in Thailand (everyday on our honeymoon at only £4 a session!) and back in the UK. It is quite a deep, intense treatment so you need to be able to stand that pressure on your feet and lower legs, but wonderfully effective for all round pain relief and deep relaxation.

CHAPTER 7:

Acupuncture

If you, like me, are a Christian, or it interests/concerns you, please also see my section on *'Considering the Spiritual Implications of alternative therapies'*.

Acupuncture is rooted in ancient Chinese medicine, and involves inserting needles into the skin at specific points of the body, along pathways called *'meridians'*. They are energy channels believed to be related to the internal organs of the body, and this energy is known as Qi. The needles are used to increase or decrease the flow of this energy, or unblock it if necessary.

I have had positive, negative and neutral experiences of acupuncture of the years. The best, by far, was through a community acupuncture clinic, where two ladies had trained in Chinese medicine, set up their own multi-bed clinic so that it could be made more affordable[17]. I was able to attend most weeks throughout studying for my degree in that town. It was on my way to college and I formed a lovely friendship with my therapist, Victoria. She was so empathetic and caring, and non judgemental, which of course could, as some believe, contribute to the effectiveness of the treatment for me.

The multi-bed treatment meant that, after a private consultation, on subsequent treatments the therapist can insert needles, leave you to rest for around 20 minutes, while they see the next patient. You are left with a bell so that you can call the therapist

---

[17]. Taunton Community Acupuncture Centre, Somerset UK. www.tauntoncommunityacupuncture.com also http://www.acmac.net is the national multi bed acupuncture association which can provide information on a centre closer to you.

at any time, and they often check in on you to make sure you are comfortable.

Acupuncture can be an incredibly effective therapy for many people, and so these clinics want to make it as accessible and affordable to people as possible. Thousands of people have found acupuncture to be effective for a variety of issues – either something specific, like arthritis in the knee, or tinnitus, or to help those who generally feel unwell yet don't have a specific diagnosis.

The treatment involved talking about symptoms and any feedback from previous sessions, whilst lying or sitting on a couch. Then fine, sterile needles are generally inserted into certain points on the body, according to which points the therapist thinks will help your symptoms. The therapist may also use things like cupping (massaging with a suction cup), oils, or an infra-red heat lamp.

> "Acupuncture focuses on the cause of disease as well as the symptoms. By addressing the underlying problem we aim to prevent future recurrences rather than merely suppressing symptoms. As a positive side effect, treatment can also boost the immune system and increase levels of energy and well-being. It can also be extremely helpful in moderating the side effects of medication[18]."

One of the benefits of acupuncture is it can be used alongside western medical treatment.

The benefits I experienced were: pain relief, improved sleep, and greatly improved digestion, to name a few. The side effects – positive mood and increased energy! I was only sad that when I moved away there were no similar clinics close by that I could afford, so I ceased to have regular acupuncture.

After having spinal surgery, I did visit a private practitioner for acupuncture, who apparently treated in the same style as Victoria. However I actually found I was in more discomfort during and after treatments, and did not attend more than 3 times, because it was also expensive. This could have been due to the fact that my recent surgery and scar tissue were just too 'raw', or that the therapist didn't quite 'click' with me, or that I was a bit more anxious about my recovery.

---

18. Victoria Watson. www.tauntoncommunityacupuncture.com

Despite Western Medicines generally non-"*alternative*" approach to treatment, acupuncture is now used in some NHS settings, such as in pain clinics or physiotherapy departments. In Western medicine, trials have found that pain messages can be stopped from reaching the brain by using acupuncture. Pain signals normally travel along a nerve to the brain, but it is possible to top that signal reaching the brain – therefore preventing the **perception** of pain.

Studies worldwide have also shown that acupuncture can release natural endorphins (natural opiates) into the nervous system, thereby giving pain relief, beyond any placebo effect. For more information on clinical studies into acupuncture read Chapter 8 in 'Healing without Freud or Prozac[19]'.

After not being able to afford private, traditional acupuncture treatment any longer, I was offered some acupuncture sessions with the physiotherapist at the hospital where I had surgery – through the NHS. The physiotherapists had basically done some extra training in 'medical acupuncture', on the premise that acupuncture can help to relieve pain by stimulating the brain and nervous system to produce pain-relieving chemicals. They do not approach it from background training in the Chinese principles of Yin, Yan and Qi, but from a more physiological perspective.

However, I found my experience of medical acupuncture very painful when they inserted the needles as well as when the needles were in, and felt bruised afterwards – a few times there were physical bruises. Perhaps the particular therapist that treated me was not very experienced or 'gifted' in the administering of needles! Or perhaps it was just a lack of traditional training and spiritual sensitivity to the treatment. Who knows?! After 6 sessions I didn't have any more. But if you are offered acupuncture for free it is worth a try.

I do not believe the original acupuncture treatment worked for me because of the placebo effect – Here's why: I was sceptical and unsure it would '*work*' initially, yet found it to be extremely beneficial. The times later when I tried it through other

---

19. For more on 'Science and Needles' see chapter 8 in 'Healing without Freud or Prozac'. Dr David Servan-Schrieber. ©2003, 2004, 2005. Rodale International Publishing.

practitioners, I then expected it to be wonderful and believed it would make me feel better – but I felt worse! Just remember, all practitioners are different.

CHAPTER 8:

Other Therapies I Have Tried

AROMATHERAPY

The ancient practice of using fragrances or oil for health benefits may help patients cope and feel better when dealing with pain and its effects on mood and stress levels. Essential oils - distracted from plants - are often diluted in a carrier oil for massage purposes, or put into something that will help disperse the scent so that it can be inhaled (e.g. an oil burner). 5-10 drops can also be added to a bath for added therapeutic effect.

Odours travel up the nose, latching onto receptors that create electrical impulses, that then travel up the olfactory nerves to the brain. It has been found that odours can change brain-wave patterns, but exactly how remains a mystery. It is known that they travel to the limbic system - where emotions and memory are processed and stored.

Whether aromatherapy *"works"* is often down to the individual experience and taste. Here are some examples of oils that are generally known to relieve stress or improve mood (and thereby perhaps lessen the intensity of pain):

ESSENTIAL OIL	USES
Basil, Rosemary, Lemon	Increase mental alertness
Lavender, Chamomile	Relieve insomnia, PMS and de-stress
Sandalwood, Geranium	Improve sex drive
Frankincense	Calm nerves

ESSENTIAL OIL	USES
Jasmine, Rose	Increase confidence
Basil, Geranium, Orange, Bergamot	Combat depression, lift mood, (I also find that bergamot can boost energy levels)
Peppermint	Soothe digestion

THE ALEXANDER TECHNIQUE

This is a postural therapy that works well in combination with other treatments and exercises. It is a method of learning to focus on how we use our body to perform our daily activities. Many of us, when undertaking everyday activities, do so with undue levels of tension which can cause pain – resulting in a stiff neck, round shoulders, lower back pain, etc..

F. M. Alexander was actually an actor who found that he was losing his voice when performing. By watching himself rehearse in the mirror and altering his stance, posture, and mindset, he was able to retrain his body to perform in a more ergonomic and relaxed fashion. A practitioner will assess you and help you sit, stand, walk, rest etc. in a more healthy efficient manner, thereby reducing unnecessary tension and pain. Hands on and verbal instruction from an Alexander technique teacher/therapist can help the individual observe their own habitual patterns and make changes where necessary in order to release tension and further postural damage. Lessons will focus on improving physical and mental well-being by reducing tension and being aware of the relationship between the head, neck and spine.

In many cultures the mind-body relationship is an intrinsic theme, but in Western society the two are often separated – which is made apparent in the extensive use of new technology, computers, television, and a general decline in physical activity. The Alexander Technique is one of the ways in which people are looking to redress the balance between mind and body[20].

---

20. For more information, see 'Alexander Technique'. A Step-by-Step Guide. Ailsa Masterton. ©Element Books Ltd 1998

BOWEN THERAPY

The Bowen Technique uses a gentle rolling action over soft tissue that intends to create a signal to the brain, based on the theory that a non intrusive treatment approach, with no adjustment or manipulation can aid balance in the body. Bowen therapy has been observed to help with pain management, including acute and chronic back pain, frozen shoulder, headaches, as well as digestive issues and chronic fatigue.

My experience of this was through the NHS with a physiotherapist who had recently trained in the Bowen Technique. I lay on my front for around 20 -30 minutes, whilst she periodically came in and lightly 'pinched' certain areas on my back. It was a little odd, and although I felt slightly relaxed (that might have been just because I was taking time out to lie down in peace and quiet!) I felt no benefit after 6 weeks of treatment, so we didn't carry on.

But like anything like this, it is worth a try with a qualified practitioner, if you can afford it.

HOMOEOPATHY

The aim of homoeopathy is to cure a disorder by treating the whole person rather than single symptoms, so the overall emotional and psychological health of the individual is regarded as significant. Homoeopaths believe that illness is a sign of imbalance within the body and that remedies prescribed should be suitable for both the symptoms, characteristics and the temperament of the patient. One remedy may also be used to treat different groups of symptoms.

Homoeopathy is based on an ancient concept that 'like produces like', formulated by Hippocrates. In the 1800s this concept was revived by Samuel Hahnemann, a German doctor. He experimented by giving minute doses of a substance that caused symptoms of an illness in a healthy person, and concluded that a diluted form of these substances could be used to fight that illness in the patient who was sick. The medicines are still used today, based on Hahnemann's work, and come from plant, mineral and animal sources. The substances are soaked in alcohol to extract the essential ingredients, and then repeatedly diluted, shaken and possibly diluted again, thought to make the properties more powerful by adding energy and removing impurities. These remedies are then made available in tablets, tinctures or ointments. There are of course many more resources for reading about homoeopathy in detail, and I have just tried to briefly explain it, if poorly!

I must admit I haven't personally had much experience with homoeopathy, and have never visited a practitioner for a one-to-one assessment treatment. I was not convinced of the efficacy of the therapy enough to pay such a fee. However the therapy has regained a huge following and respect in the 20th century and many more conventional therapists might incorporate the use of homoeopathy in their treatment approaches.

ARNICA
I have used the homeopathic remedy Arnica repeatedly for pain related to bruising or tissue damage – such as post surgery and post childbirth, or falling and hurting my back in a 'bruised' kind of way. I do believe it aids the natural healing process. Arnica is available in tiny tablets which you place under your tongue every few hours for a certain amount of time (follow the instructions on the bottle) and can be purchased at most good chemists. I have also purchased massage oil containing arnica, or a more concentrated form of arnica massage balm – this has also been useful for things like strained wrists or carpal tunnel syndrome.

CHAPTER 9:

Magnetic Therapy

Magnetic therapy is an alternative practice that uses static magnets to alleviate pain or some other health problem. So-called therapeutic magnets are typically integrated into bracelets, (often copper bracelets for which you may have seen adverts in alternative health magazines) necklaces, or shoe inserts, as well as magnetic mattresses, back or joint supports, and chair pads.

The most common suggested mechanism is that magnets might improve blood flow in underlying tissues. However, those who have looked at it scientifically would say that the field surrounding magnet therapy devices is said to be far too weak and falls off with distance far too quickly to appreciably affect blood components, muscles, bones, blood vessels, or organs.

> 'Many well-conducted studies over the past three decades have shown that static magnetic devices offer no more or no less benefit than sham devices devoid of a magnet. These studies suggest that static magnetic therapy devices may not work at all beyond having a placebo effect on those who wear them.'

Despite a lack of scientific evidence to support claims that magnetic therapy devices work, wearable magnets remain extremely popular. When I lived in the States, I became friends with a couple who sold magnetic healing devices, as part of a home-based business linked with the franchise company Nikken[22]. They were so enthusiastic and convinced that their

---

21. www.livescience.com/40174-magnetic-therapy.html
22. www.nikken.com

products would heal me, and I of course was taken in by this, having only been suffering for around 4 years and still very open minded to try anything.

The first Nikken product, the Magstep®, was an insole to help people with aching and tired feet and the negative affects this had on the body. The inspiration for the energizing massage nodes on the insoles was derived from the pebbled surface at the bottom of a Japanese public bath. They added magnetism to the insoles to intensify the field of energy.

I tried the Magstep, and believed they really worked to help me walk more, decrease back pain, and give me energy. Whether or not it was the placebo effect, I can't be sure. I went on to purchase a very expensive chair pad, since sitting was when I experienced the most pain, and I needed to sit in order to study, attend church and college, do art, work at the computer, etc.. I took that seat pad everywhere with me for quite some time. But whether or not it was the magnets, or the supportive cushion shape that helped, or simply that I believed it would help because my friends said it would, and I had paid a lot of money for it, I can't be sure!

I tried out magnetic bracelets, copper bracelets with magnets in them, neck supports, wraps for my back, and even bought an even more expensive portable device that was some sort of wonder-machine that had spinning high powered magnets inside, and if I simply aimed it at the area of pain, it was supposed to effect change inside my body within minutes! I can't even remember what happened to that, to be honest. I don't think I would buy another magnetic product, but don't let me stop you trying if you wish to.

CHAPTER 10:

Considering the Spiritual Implications of Alternative Therapies

Certain therapies may have spiritual roots that make their pursuit inappropriate for Christians. With a plethora of alternative therapies on offer, if you are a Christian you may be thinking about how to evaluate your therapy choices based on Biblical advice, and making sure you are not getting involved in any treatment that uses, or is based on, a spirituality that is contrary to God's will for us. Some alternative therapies are based on practices and rituals that have been a part of pagan traditions or other religious practices, and the spiritual basis of a therapy can be an important concept to consider.

We should investigate claims made about remedies we put in our bodies, or practitioners whom we allow to treat us.

> "Do you not know that your body is a temple of the Holy Spirit, who is in you, who you have received from God? You are not your own; you were bought at a high price. Therefore honour God with your body".
> 1 Corinthians 6:19-20

One resource I must acknowledge in thinking about these issues for myself, and writing this book, is 'Alternative Medicine, The Christian Handbook[23]', which I will refer to, but also encourage you to read it yourself for much more information on the spiritual background of therapies I have not covered in this book, and scriptures to help you make informed, God-honouring

---

23. 'Alternative Medicine, The Christian Handbook', Donal O'Mathuna, Ph.D. & Walt Larimore, M.D. Published by Zondervan. ©2001.

decisions regarding your treatment. The book is endorsed by the Christian Medical Association (CMA) which is a movement to help Christian health care professionals integrate their faith and professional practice.

Not all alternative therapies are rooted in a religious tradition, but some are – such as those rooted in Wiccan (white witchcraft), life energy channels, or shamanism. Holistic medicine can include the acceptance of all things spiritual – and some people claim this spirituality can be whatever the individual wants it to mean. But the Bible tells us not to engage in certain practices, because they use prohibited methods, and can ultimately lead people away from the one true God. Prohibited are such things as divination, mediumship, witchcraft, magic, and sorcery, and some of these have been incorporated into certain alternative therapies, even though it may not seem obvious to us.

An alternative therapy using contact with any spirit other than God is forbidden for Christians – e.g. shamanism, reiki, channelling, and tarot cards. The book I mentioned above discusses this in much more detail and for that reason I will not go into it too much here.

It is helpful to ask yourself *'What Spiritual beliefs and values underlie the therapy or are held by the therapist?'*

It is true that some people practicing acupuncture base their practice on ancient Chinese Medicine, and therefore the principles of manipulating life energy. Yet I do not personally say that means Christians should have nothing to do with acupuncture, because I believe it works in purely physical ways and healing systems which God himself created in our bodies. *'Just because some people use acupuncture needles to manipulate life energy does not automatically mean Christians should have nothing to do with acupuncture. A remedy may be acceptable if the physical components can be separated from the underlying belief system, analogous to how Paul separated the meat from the idolatry*[24]*'.* In 1 Corinthians 8 - 10 Christians were debating whether they should eat meat sold in the marketplace that had originally been sacrificed to idols in pagan temples. They were concerned that

---

24. Donal O'Mathuna, Ph.D. & Walt Larimore, M.D. ©2001 'Alternative Medicine, The Christian Handbook', published by Zondervan. p. 76

they were connecting themselves with occult activities. However Paul advised them to eat any meat sold in the market with a clear conscience, quoting *"The earth is the Lord's, and everything in it."*

In investigating any therapy for yourself, I definitely encourage you to pray for personal conviction and guidance either way, to look to the Bible, and to do more research.

The only other therapy I have tried that seems to have a grey area around its acceptance among Christians is yoga. I have found yoga to be of great benefit in releasing back pain and preventing more pain on that day and days afterward. I use it to stretch out muscles of my body that need working and stretching – thereby taking care of the body God gave me – preventing more pain and building strength, and using the breathing techniques to relax and release muscle tension. However, I prefer to practice it at home alone, and if I attend a class I am careful to select one that does not involve any alternative spiritual practices or a teacher who might engage in those.

I would stay away from those practitioners who encourage poses held to promote meditation to *'bring me in touch with my inner voice'*. The Bible teaches that human nature (and therefore our own inner voice) is not divine or perfect, whereas New Age beliefs hold that human nature is good and perfect – even divine.

Yoga is rooted in Eastern religions. The word yoga literally means 'union', and the practice is integral to the Hindu religion where it implies union with the 'divine', and aims to bring spiritual enlightenment. However, still there are many who practice or teach yoga that view it simply as a set of breathing and stretching exercises, designed to improve strength, relaxation, and thus health. It is best, as a Christian, to choose a form of exercise and relaxation that has no spiritual underpinnings, but some forms of yoga, or some poses, can be helpful to release and prevent physical pain, so I just adopt those physical elements into my own exercise regime.

Meditation is another element of many alternative therapies, and which often has spiritual roots contrary to the Bible. While I don't meditate, as such, I do engage in contemplative prayer and listening out for the Holy Spirit's voice whilst stretching or relaxing. I find meditative Christian music or good classical music can aid this and keep me focused on why I am there – to stretch, relax, and connect with God.

Qigong emphasises the importance of taking time to relax and do gentle exercise, but along with Tai Chi, is also designed to help people become more unified with a universal energy or *'Universal Consciousness'*. Also, some Qigong masters claim to have paranormal activities that indicate they may be tapping into some psychic or spiritual power, other than God.

Christians should indeed take a holistic approach to their health – taking time to exercise, relax, reduce stress, etc., but it is easy to do that without engaging in practices that are infused with non-Christian concepts. If there is an exercise class offered simply that utilises the physically beneficial techniques of Tai Chi or Qigong, without a teacher who is immersed in the religious backgrounds and beliefs of the practice, I would personally be willing to try it. These forms of exercise are said to have many general health benefits, such as lowering blood pressure, tension, easing depression, fatigue, anxiety, and improving digestion and circulation.

Reflexology came to be a named therapy in the 20th Century, based on the belief that energy flows through various zones in the body and must be balanced in order for organs in that zone to be healthy. Reflex points (generally on the feet) connected with that zone are massaged to rebalance the energy and allegedly restore health. Some practitioners claim reflexology works by improving the blood flow to the corresponding parts of the body, and aiding detoxification. Other practitioners utilize the more spiritual concept of life energy, as in the Chinese *'Chi'* or Indian *'Prana'*.

Reflexology does seem to aid relaxation, but be careful of the potential for life energy involvement. An ordinary foot massage could be just as beneficial.

Before trying any of these therapies, investigate them, find out what spiritual roots exist, find out where the practitioner or teacher is coming from in the spiritual sense, find out what teaching you will be exposed to, talk to wise and discerning Christian leaders, and pray about it.

'Taking charge of the areas of your health that you can control helps to optimize how you feel even in the midst of the aches and pains of fibromyalgia'

Harris H. McIlwain, M.D. and Debra Fulghum Bruce, PhD
The Fibromyalgia Handbook. Copyright 1996. Holt Paperback. p204

SECTION III

More Practical Self Management

CHAPTER 11:

Nutrition and Supplements

Eating a healthy balanced diet low in fat, refined sugar and high in antioxidants and phytochemicals (found in plant foods) helps to boost the body's immune system and promote energy and alertness – essential in chronic pain conditions which are usually accompanied by lethargy and fatigue.

Nutrients are compounds in foods that support the body's repair, growth and wellness, and include vitamins, minerals, proteins, carbohydrates, water, and essential fats. Some of these nutrients are made by the body, and others have to be provided by diet or supplementation, to prevent deficiencies leading to illness.

There is an inexhaustible amount of material in the world already written on diet and nutrition for various ailments as well as for general health or weight management. Ongoing research can cause professional opinions to change, and advice in the media is often changing and conflicting, causing much confusion about what is the best eating plan to follow, or which new life-changing dietary supplements to spend our money on.

Add to that the fact that individuals may have varying intolerances and reactions to certain foods that others don't have. For instance, after years of trying various and drastic elimination diets, my father learned that his arthritis only flared up with red meat and vegetables from the nightshade family, and he was cured as long as he did not eat these foods. After years in my childhood suffering colic and abdominal pain I discovered it was pasteurised and processed dairy products which were the culprit, and after the age of 18 I found myself excessively more tired and bloated when I consume wheat or gluten.

So here I will just share some general points relevant to pain and fibromyalgia that I have found helpful or interesting and that might help you. It will require educating yourself a little about nutrition and then exercising self discipline and effort to make any necessary changes in your diet.

NEUROTRANSMITTERS, PAIN, AND NUTRITION

Certain foods affect not only our digestive system but also our brain chemistry, and brain chemistry is directly linked with our perception of physical pain, energy levels, and our mood. Food is one of the most powerful tools for changing brain chemistry.

Serotonin is a feel-good neurotransmitter associated with the feelings of relaxation, lessened anxiety, the ability to concentrate, and optimism; serotonin elevates mood and plays a role in fibromyalgia symptoms – especially those with depression and sleep problems. Eaten in moderation, the high complex carbohydrate foods can help boost serotonin levels, e.g. bread, pasta, potatoes, rice.

On the other hand, high protein foods such as chicken, turkey, tuna or other proteins can help boost attention and energy levels – those foods rich in an amino acid called tyrosine. When we eat high protein foods, this increases the levels of tyrosine, which boosts levels of the neurotransmitters dopamine and norepinephrine – which make us more alert, energetic, assertive and able to concentrate. It is recommended to include a protein source in our diets several times a day.

Too little protein in the diet can lead to fatigue, lethargy, weakness and poor immunity. There are ways vegetarians can substitute with non-animal proteins when they combine them with certain complementary starches. E.g. beans with bread, legumes with grains.

For more information about the relationship between neurochemistry and diet and lifestyle I highly recommend reading *'Natural Prozac – Learning to Release Your Body's own Anti-Depressants'*, by Dr. Joel Roberston with Tom Monte. Copyright 1997. HarperCollins. It is an excellent resource on explaining depression and neurochemicals, and how diet, exercise, thinking, and things like music and other activities can be used for self-management. Since physical pain and low mood often co-exist, I have found this book to be very informative and helpful, whilst being easy to understand. There is also more on neurochemistry and the links with pain in chapter 4.

CAFFEINE
Caffeine is a stimulant and should be avoided, especially after mid-afternoon, if you struggle with sleeping well at night. This can be hard to avoid completely, especially waking up with 'fibro-fog' or when taking medications that cause drowsiness. Because of this I find I do need some caffeine to function and work, and especially to exercise – which is essential for pain management, but I don't overdose on caffeine and don't have any after 4pm if I want to sleep that night.

ALCOHOL
I have to admit that I am quite partial to a glass or 2 of wine in the evenings, particularly when pain feels unmanageable and I need to relax! Of course I can't say this is advisable, and it can add to more sleep disturbance and morning 'fogginess' and fatigue for some people. There is a herbal supplement that I take when I drink alcohol, called Milk Thistle, which helps the liver do its job of detoxifying. As long as you also drink plenty of water before going to sleep, the unpleasant effects of an occasional drink or two can be eliminated. Moderation is key. And self discipline or even further support is needed if you are prone to wanting to block out the pain on a regular basis in this way.

NUTRITIONAL SUPPLEMENTS
All of the essential nutrients we need in our body (those we don't make ourselves but must provide through diet) are not always provided by our modern diets or absorbed enough by the body. Therefore for all-round health, it is a good practice to take a supplement containing all the essential vitamins and minerals, especially if your immune system is compromised or you don't feel you have a healthy diet. No specific evidence favours some more than others for chronic pain issues, so for a better chance at achieving balanced nutrition, take a supplement containing them all! (according to the RDA suggested).

MORE PRACTICAL SELF MANAGEMENT | 81

Vitamin D is essential for the production of serotonin - the feelgood neurochemical (see chapter 4) and although you can get this in a supplement, it is best manufactured in the body by getting out into sunlight at least 2-3 times a week, to boost supplies.

Iron is especially important for the production of energy in the body, preventing or treating fatigue caused by an iron deficiency. Make sure your diet contains iron rich foods such as apricots, lean red meats, beans, lentils, prunes or raisins. To boost the absorption of iron in the body it is important to consume it alongside a food rich in vitamin C (or a supplement).

Evidence suggests that the B vitamins may help to alleviate some fibromyalgia symptoms. E.g. Folic acid seems to help with mood management. One 8 week study of 213 patients with depression found that those with low folic acid levels were less likely to respond to treatment with fluoxetine (Prozac), an antidepressant medication commonly used for fibromyalgia patients.[25] (I personally have been prescribed fluoxetine for many years now, both for my mood and pain levels, and have experienced major drops in my ability to cope with both factors each time I have tried to come off the medication, so I know that for me, it is a medication I need to help support my brain chemistry functioning as well as it can.)

Vitamin B12 is also said to help with memory function, nerve damage, muscle weakness, and fatigue. 'I include this chart (on the following page) from my well-used book, *'The Fibromyalgia Handbook26'* to help you include B vitamins in your diet:'

---

25. Research quoted in Harris H.McIlwain, M.D. and Debra Fulghum Bruce, Ph.D The Fibromyalgia Handbook. Copyright 1996. Holt Paperbacks p. 209
26. The 'Fibromyalgia Handbook'. P. 209

FOOD SOURCES OF THERAPEUTIC B VITAMINS	
B1 (Thiamine)	Wheat germ, peanuts, peas
B2 (Riboflavin)	Dairy produce, broccoli, tuna, salmon
B3 (Niacin)	Brewers yeast (Marmite!) poultry, eggs, peanuts
B6 (Pyridoxine)	Soy beans, liver, fish, bananas, oatmeal
B12 (Colabamine)	Oysters, eggs, dairy products
Folic Acid	Green leafy vegetables, asparagus, cantaloupe, spinach, lima beans, tofu, sweet potatoes, citrus fruits, peanuts
Biotin	Liver, nuts, legumes, egg yolks
Pantothenic acid	Cheese, cauliflower, beans, sweet potatoes

When buying supplements do go for reputable brands, rather than a cheap supermarket-own brand or one from a pound shop, to ensure they are of a decent quality and therefore more likely to be absorbed and used effectively in the body.

Having said all this, these supplements are not to replace the need to eat as healthy and balanced a diet as possible, but to *'supplement'* it, as the name suggests.

MAGNESIUM

Deficiencies of this mineral have been found to be associated with chronic pain conditions such as fibromyalgia in clinical studies. Magnesium is vital for muscle health and deficiencies can be experienced as muscle tension, spasms, and restlessness. Studies now show that magnesium is important for inhibiting nerve receptors linked to pain trigger points; 500mg of oral magnesium taken daily was shown to influence fibromyalgia symptoms[27], as well as alleviate menstrual cramps.

Foods to be included in the diet containing significant levels of magnesium include nuts, sunflower seeds, cereals, barley, quinoa, tofu, dairy products, bananas, avocados, spinach, oysters, mackerel, cod.

I have recently been trying a product called 'Better You Magnesium Oil Spray' that you spray directly onto the painful muscle area and rub in. I particularly wanted to try it for my neck and shoulder spasms. It claims that when spraying this essential mineral directly into the skin tissue, it efficiently replaces magnesium faster than an oral supplementation. I had read anecdotal reports of it helping pain in magazine articles and quotes from medical doctors on some websites that claim it can bring pain relief and muscle relaxation for people with arthritis and muscle cramping. I am sure that combined with a professional massage, on a regular basis, it would increase magnesium levels in the body and hopefully reduce muscle cramping. But so far, simply using it at home, applying the recommended 10 sprays to the affected area when it is in spasm, I have not noticed much change. Perhaps I need to try it for longer and more frequently, which would require me spending more money on a larger bottle.

OMEGA 3 FATTY ACIDS

Some foods are known to decrease inflammation in the body. Omega 3 fatty acids are one of these foods and the best sources can be found in fish such as tuna and mackerel, or fish oils. Supplements of Omega 3 fish oil come in capsules or liquid, or you can get vegetarian alternatives derived from flax seed oil or evening primrose oil. (I actually also take evening primrose oil and swear by its positive effects on female monthly hormonal symptoms).

The reports of omega 3 supplementation helping the symptoms of arthritic type pain are mostly anecdotal, but I have read enough over the years to convince me to try it and I now have been taking it regularly for a few years. I can only say that when

27. Alternative Medicine Alert Journal March 2002.

I have gone through a month or so of forgetting to take it, or getting out of the habit of taking it, it has seemed to me that I have experienced more pain in my joints. Scientific studies of fibromyalgia patients taking the supplements have not yet been conclusive, but perhaps they have not been carried out extensively enough. Taken in the recommended dosage, it can do no harm to the body, and there are also claims it can help with brain function and patients with depression. A diet rich in omega 3 fish oils leads, in the long run, to an increased production of neurotransmitters in the brain for energy and positive mood, and there is much interesting evidence on the implications of using these nutrients to help manage mental health issues[28].

MILK THISTLE

If you take medications or drink occasionally, toxins can build up in the liver, and this herb can help the liver to detoxify itself. But do not think this replaces the well known importance of drinking plenty of water and eating plenty of fresh fruit and vegetables.

PROBIOTICS

I am throwing this one in for anyone who may also suffer with digestive problems or food intolerances. Since taking probiotics (as well as following a healthy diet) I have had much healthier gut with so much less colic/wind symptoms, healthy bowel movements and almost no bloating. I used to suffer on a daily basis with these things throughout my teenage years and early 20s, and found that although wheat and some dairy products were the main culprits, probiotics helped my gut heal so that when I do now have these just occasionally, I don't suffer the consequences. Also, having taken medications for many years that can have effect the lining of the stomach and cause digestive discomfort; probiotics have again been my friend in healing and preventing further problems. Although there are many probiotic drinks on the market, to get the maximum dose and benefit, I recommend taking a supplement available from a reputable health food store, and be sure not to take it with hot food or

---

28. See chapter 9 'The Revolution in Nutrition: Omega 3 Fatty Acids Feed the Emotional Brain' in 'Healing without Freud or Prozac' Dr David Servan-Schrieber. ©2003, 2004, 2005. Rodale International Publishing.

drink (the healthy bacteria are destroyed by heat before being able to reach your gut).

PEPPERMINT OIL CAPSULES

For the same problems of digestion discussed above, and particularly with medications that have a negative side effect on the stomach/bowel, I have made these a staple ingredient in my cupboard or to have with me when travelling. I like eating healthy meals, as well as the odd treat, and I hate the pain of trapped wind or indigestion. I can literally feel these soothing a sore tummy when I need to take one.

OTHER SUPPLEMENTS RECOMMENDED THAT I HAVE TRIED

5-HTP

5-Hydroxytryptophan (5-HTP) is a compound derived from tryptophan and is used to increase the synthesis of serotonin in the central nervous system. Tryptophan is converted to 5-HTP in the body which can then be converted into serotonin. One study reported that supplementation of 5-HTP eased depression, anxiety and insomnia, as well as somatic pains in those with fibromyalgia. Yet some studies show no benefit at all. This supplement is available from good health food stores if you want to give it a try - I have done so, but noticed no benefit as of yet.

GINSENG

Ginseng is said to boost mental and physical performance and alertness, so I have bought a pot of these supplements quite frequently in the hope of feeling less fatigued and not feeling the need for caffeine. There are few different types available – Siberian ginseng, Korean Ginseng. Personally I have not noticed any significant benefit from taking these supplements, but give them a try for yourself.

ALOE VERA JUICE

There are many claims that this super plant food can boost health and even cure many symptoms of ill health. I think every health food journal or shop has material promoting its benefits and trying to sell the various products containing Aloe Vera. I was taken in by the Forever Living Company's claims of health obtained by drinking the juice on a daily basis, however I experienced no noticeable benefit, and it tasted fowl! Perhaps that was just me. There must be something good in it or so many people would not claim it so?

DEVILS CLAW

This is a herbal remedy said to help with back pain in particular. The native African plant gets its name because the fruit is covered with hooks meant to attach onto animals in order to spread the seeds. The roots and tubers of the plant are used to make medicine. For years I was put off by the title, but did give it a go some time ago. Again, I can't say I noticed any benefit even though I took the maximum recommended dose over a number of months. Other reports and even scientific studies have shown some benefit for those taking Devils Claw who have low back pain or osteoarthritis, even lowering the dose of NSAIDS needed. Perhaps it works in a similar way, and I don't really respond to NSAIDS, so it may be worth trying for yourself if your problem is associated with inflammatory pain. For other symptoms, Devils Claw has not been shown to significantly help.

MELATONIN

This hormone is available over-the-counter in supplement form, although melatonin is a natural hormone that helps to set the brain's body clock, which determines all of the body's circadian rhythms - including hormone release, temperature, sleep cycles, and digestion. As a supplement, the advice is to take it one or two hours before bedtime, not during the daytime. Do talk to your Dr before trying it, as with any supplements. You may find it helps regulate your sleep and wake cycle in a more natural way than sedatives would. I have tried it many years ago, in particular when travelling (for jet lag), and found it somewhat effective, although I did not use it long-term.

GLUCOSAMINE/CHONDROTIN/MSM
In the early days of experiencing back and join pain, not knowing the causes, I experimented with taking supplements such as those that many people with arthritis use to ease pain. Glucosamine and chondroitin are common examples, and some have added Methyl sulfonylmethane (MSM). Glucosamine and chondroitin sulfate are the building blocks for cartilage and appear to stimulate the body to make more cartilage. There are conflicting studies on glucosamine and chondroitin, some demonstrating a beneficial effect on osteoarthritis pain. Research is ongoing, but many physicians may still recommend a trial of glucosamine at this point, and if there is not apparent improvement by three months, it would be reasonable to stop glucosamine.

MSM, is a chemical found naturally in plants, animals, and humans, or manufactured synthetically, and many people use MSM as a medicine. MSM is actually a type of sulfur supplement; It's been suggested to cure arthritis, chronic joint pain, and similar diseases.

SULFUR
There are two types of sulfur supplements: MSM and sulfur. When I first visited a chiropractor, she also gave me sulphur supplements and recommended I take a compound of glucosamine/chondroitin/MSM, but I was never quite sure why.

All MSM contains sulfur, but not all sulfur contains MSM, which is simply a naturally-occurring compound produced by most living creatures – so it's one of the easiest forms of sulfur to access for those who have been recommended it to heal common aches and pains. Some people take sulphur in the form of MSM regularly to treat conditions like arthritis, rheumatoid arthritis, and osteoarthritis, where it's been suggested to reduce stiffness, improve flexibility, and reduce pain.

Here are some of the supposed benefits of sulfur:

·Sulfur is thought to be a powerful antioxidant because it encourages the body's natural production of glutathione, which is one of the body's most important antioxidants. Without sulfur, your body can't produce glutathione.

·Sulfur is one of the building blocks for amino acids (and thus protein). Without sulfur, your body can't produce amino acids, which are especially important for promoting lean muscle growth.

·Sulfur is thought to reduce bone and joint pain by acting as a calcium phosphate dissolver. Thus, it breaks down unhealthy calcium deposits throughout the body.

·Improve Skin and Hair Health

·Acts as a Natural Energy Booster

> 'Out of all the benefits listed here, this is the benefit backed by the least amount of science. Some people take sulfur as a natural energy booster. The idea is that sulfur will increase the permeability of the cell membrane, which means cells need less energy to expel toxins. When cells can more easily expel toxins, it means they have more energy to digest food and turn that into physical and mental energy[29]'.

Ultimately, there have been no reputable scientific reports or clinical tests involving humans and sulfur, and so the benefits are unproven. If you read a reference to some *"groundbreaking"* sulfur study, it was most likely performed on animals and not humans.

Sulfur and MSM can be found in almost all raw foods. Here are some of the surprising natural food sources of sulfur:

Leafy Green Vegetables
Beer And Coffee
Raw Milk
Eggs
Meats, Poultry, And Fish
Soy Products, Legumes, Nuts, Seeds, And Grains
Asparagus, Brussels Sprouts, Garlic, Onions, Kale, And Wheat Germ
B Vitamins
All Fruits

There's a reason sulfur deficiency isn't common: it's in almost every food we eat, and is produced in our bodies every day anyway. Cooking processes can greatly reduce MSM levels in food. If you want to maximize the amount of sulfur in your diet, you should focus on eating raw fruits and vegetables.[30]

NADH

NADH, or reduced nicotinamide adenine dinucleotide, is a naturally occuring enzyme (made from niacin, a B Vitamin) in all living cells which helps produce energy. Some patients with CFS / ME showed promising results - notably less fatigue, and more mental and physical energy. Because there are many people that have overlapping symptoms of Chronic Fatigue Syndrome and Fibromyalgia, I have included this interesting information here.

The NY Daily News and other publications reported that 72% of the patients in a CFS study experienced and reported positive improvements when taking 10mg of NADH daily. Dr Birkmayer, (the Doctor that developed stabilized NADH) recommends 60mg to 80mg of NADH daily to recognize better results or quicker results than those obtained in the clinical studies[31].

The use of NADH in fibromyalgia is based more on 'anecdotal evidence and hypothetical matches between the supplement's known functions and the conditions' known deficiencies and symptoms. As a coenzyme, NADH helps enzymes in your body break down food and convert it to energy in the form of adenosine triphosphate (ATP).

Research also shows that NADH can stimulate brain function, which may help alleviate the cognitive dysfunction associated with FMS and ME/CFS. NADH may reduce the fatigue of chronic disease by restoring function of the mitochondria (tiny structures that power your cells.) Fatigue is a major symptom of both FMS and ME/CFS.

NADH may help your brain create neurotransmitters that may be deficient in these conditions (serotonin, norepinephrine, and dopamine.)

29. & 30. Notes on Sulphur and MSM derived from supplementpolice.com/sulfur-supplements/
31. nadh.com/pages/cfs

We have no research on it for FMS. Limited research shows that NADH may be an effective treatment for ME/CFS and also depression, Parkinson's disease, and Alzheimer's disease. However, more study is needed before we can say how effective a treatment it is for any illnesses[32'].

---

32. www.verywell.com/nadh-for-fibromyalgia-chronic-fatigue-syndrome-715795

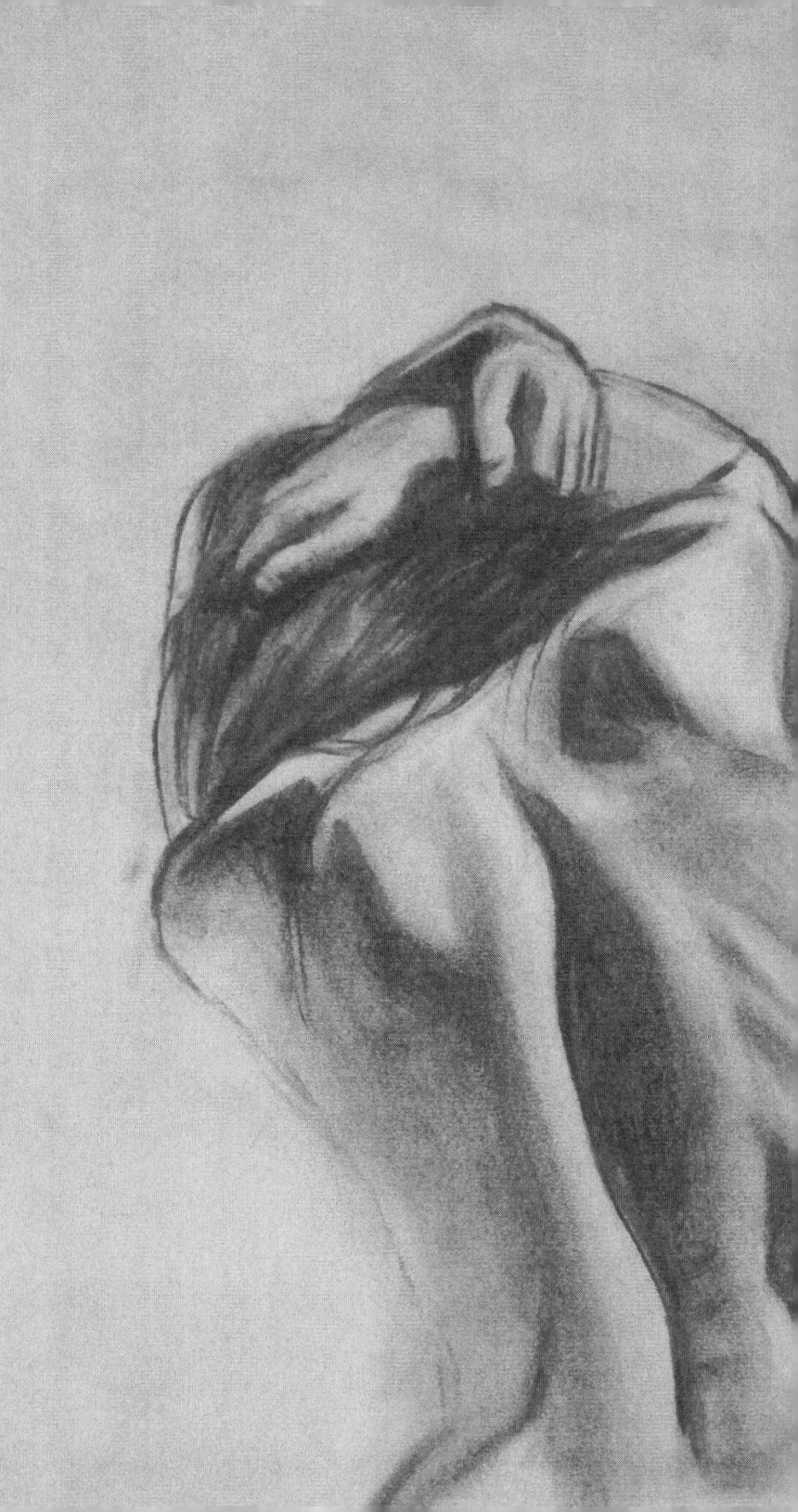

CHAPTER 12:

Sleep

Restorative sleep is imperative. It is vital for everyone – but especially those with chronic pain, fibromyalgia, arthritic conditions, ME/CFS or the like, to get a decent and comfortable nights rest – or at least as much as possible! Yet pain affects your ability to sleep, and the lack of sleep makes the pain seem worse and helps create the constant state of fatigue many sufferers experience.

> "Pain can be the main reason that someone wakes up multiple times a night, and this results in a decrease in sleep quantity and quality, and on the flip side, sleep deprivation can lower your pain threshold and pain tolerance and make existing pain feel worse."

It is an ongoing reality for me that poor sleep leads to more pain and fatigue, which leads to more need for painkillers, caffeine, stress, not sleeping well again, being reliant on sleeping pills, and it becomes a vicious circle. Some researches even believe that fibromyalgia may be caused by long-term non-restorative sleep, and scientists have discovered abnormal amounts of the alpha activity on the brain scans of fibromyalgia patients during their sleep cycles. Alpha activity in the brain is associated with feeling calm and serene. Fibromyalgia symptoms have even been induced in healthy volunteers who were deprived of sleep. "Fibrofog" is a term you may have come across, and describes the fuzziness, forgetfulness, and inability to concentrate many patients struggle with, even causing them to have to give up their jobs.

Artwork, 'Pain & Beauty' by Amy Jo Haskins (Samuel). Graphite & Charcoal. 2017 www.amyjo-arts.co.uk

I have tried many mattresses and pillows over the years, trying to find the perfect type for maximum rest and comfort. But of course everyone is different and I can't say one type is best for all. For me, it is an original Temper mattress. And if not, then memory foam toppers on a general orthopedic mattress. Visit bed shops and try many out - lie on them in the store for as long as you can without feeling self conscious!

Recently a specialist spinal physiotherapist asked how my sleep patterns are. I had to admit that I cannot remember a time when I did not struggle with getting regular, restful sleep – it must have been when I was a child. He explained how chronic sleep problems, and especially those like sleep Apnea, can lead to the body experiencing chronic pain that is neurological by nature –i.e. it is not due to a mechanical dysfunction, but to overactive and dysfunctional pain signals in the nervous system – but of course felt by us in the muscles or joints. Treating sleep problems is a big part of managing conditions like fibromyalgia.

I am obviously no expert on this! But there are many books, alternative therapies, even courses and online apps to help you tackle your sleep disorder, if you have one. Also of course talk to your health professional, bearing in mind that a GP might prescribe tranquilizers or a milder sleep medication, which can become addictive and not really deal with the underlying problem. They can be helpful for short term sleep problems however.

CHAPTER 13:

Other Helpful Devices

One very helpful pain relief device that I must also mention here is a Tens Machine, as well as the use of hot and cold packs - please see my section on the use of these in the chapter on Physiotherapy p. 21.

As a back pain sufferer, somewhere along the line I heard about the *'The Back Show'* - held in London or Birmingham, where providers of therapies, gadgets and gizmos to help relieve pain, all congregate to exhibit and try and sell you their live-changing product. (Sorry if there is an element of cynicism in my tone!) It is actually a really interesting visit and informative visit, and can instill hope if you dare to believe in some of the products and treatments being demonstrated.

The UK's national back pain charity Back Care now organize the show, and you can register for free entry on their website[34] and find out more details about the annual show. The Back Care charity produce a quarterly magazine, as well as helpful information sheets, all available on their website, or you can read back-copies online as well[35].

The show is rather large, so if you struggle to get around or get overwhelmed and fatigued, it is worth spending 2 days to go through it, or take a wheelchair and carer if you can. They usually have scheduled exercise demos/classes as well so you can try sessions like Pilates or tai chi. Also there are scheduled seminars from spinal surgeons, top physiotherapists and the

34. www.thebackpainshow.co.uk
35. www.backcare.org.uk

like, presenting new and latest research, so these are really worth attending, but you may need to book in advance if you want to sit down!

As well as trying out some therapies – which I will give mention later, here are some of the things I decided to invest in from the show:

AN INVERSION TABLE

Traction inversion tables are for the patient to use at home, to help restore alignment of the spine. Traction - refers to the mechanism of straightening bones and relieving pressure on the spine and skeletal system. Basically you lie on the table and then *'hang'* upside down or somewhere in between, for a few minutes a day. When the body is inverted and the weight is suspended from the lower body, the pull of gravity decompresses the joints of the spine and body - in theory relieving the pressure on the discs and nerves.

I tried this out at the show a few times, to be sure it *'felt'* good, before investing in the Teeter hang up inversion table. I have to say, it did help relieve lower back pain and help me feel stretched out and relieve the pressure on my spine. I used it quite regularly, to the amusement of my housemates who would come in and find me, hanging like a bat, in the basement! Since I knew part of the problem with my back was compression in the lower spine, it made sense to try and use something to reverse this pressure.

The only reason I am not using the inversion table today, is because it is not recommended for those with metal implants in their spine, and I had bought this before having the spinal surgery. It helped, it didn't cure, and I would recommend it if you do not have metal in your spine and you feel like your lower back pain would be helped by your spine being *'opened'* up and allowed to stretch and breathe. When the discs are decompressed, nutrients can flow in via interspinal fluids, rehydrating and nourishing the spinal system.

There are likely other companies that make inversion tables, but I have just included one for reference.[36] If you get to attend the Back Show, it is best to try these out before you buy.

---

36. For more about Teeter hang-up systems, see teeter-online.co.uk

SPECIALIST PILLOWS

If you have back pain or fibromyalgia, you will probably also experience occasional or frequent neck and shoulder pain. It is crucial that when you are in bed, you are comfortable and supported in the best way possible so that your muscles and joints can relax and repair. You may have already tried many pillows and found them too soft, too hard, too flat, too deep... I'm afraid there is no perfect pillow that suits everyone and you may just have to try out a few that look like they might suit you, even if it costs money. I have bought various ones over the years, including contoured ones and memory foam ones, and felt that they helped for a while but then needed to be changed a few months later. They can also feel different depending on what mattress you are lying on underneath.

Go to a good bed shop and try lying on the beds whilst trying out various pillows they have on sale. Many will sell the Tempur ones, their own memory foam brand, or just basic feather pillows. This is something you will just have to try out until you find the one that gives you most comfort.

A PUTNAM WEDGE

A wedged cushion may help some people with back pain, particularly when sitting. The main one I know of and have tried is the Putnam Wedge, which adapts a horizontal seat to an angle, gently rocking the pelvis forward on the hips, thereby hopefully taking the strain off the lower back. For my particular problem I did not find this helpful or comfortable, but take some advice from your physiotherapist or chiropractor, and see if you can use one on trial before buying.

LUMBAR SUPPORTS AND CHAIRS

There are so many back supports on the market designed to relieve pressure on certain parts of the spine when sitting in chairs that are not designed well ergonically... lumbar rolls, for example can be helpful to keep a natural curve in the spine whilst seated. Sometimes simply rolling up a towel or blanket to use in the small of your back can help. If I am out at a coffee shop or restaurant and forgot to bring a cushion, I might roll up my coat or scarf to act as a back support, and I try to avoid stools wherever possible. Although if you have just occasional back pain, it can be a good discipline to sit on a stool and hold proper posture, without straining. I just find I cannot do this for long without causing more pain, and although I did not, many sufferers of mild back pain find the kneeling posture stools are helpful, particularly for office work.

Something as simple as a mesh lumbar support may be comfortable for you and is available online or I actually bought mine in Asda! Do ask your physiotherapist for advice on what supports might help you.

It goes without saying that posture is KEY when dealing with pain in the back, neck, shoulders, etc.. Do have a physiotherapist or Alexander Technique practitioner assess your postural habits. A good Pilates teacher is also very helpful for one-to-one sessions on correcting your posture and teaching you how to move and exercise properly.

It is absolutely essential that as much as possible when you are seated, your chair is supportive and helps you sit with good postural form and without slouching or straining. I have a specialized office chair that I use for most things as I work from home, but I was lucky enough to get funding for that when I was at university. Many towns have specialist shops for chairs and furniture for people with back pain – showing how common it is! Do go and try some out. For some people, a well designed office chair is adequate.

Small cushions or lumbar supports can also be added to chairs/sofas or carried around in the car for restaurants and visiting friends etc.. I have never been able to sit comfortably on a sofa, even though I have shopped around. I do get on well with the Poang chair from Ikea.

CHAPTER 14:

Pregnancy and Childbirth

I always guessed these two things would be challenging for someone with chronic pain and fatigue, but as long as my spinal surgeon thought it was safe, it didn't put me off trying. It could have, and I'll admit there have been days when I have not felt well enough to look after a child – so I have help, but I do not regret my decision to have children.

One of the first things to consider when trying to conceive (or as soon as you find out you are pregnant) is to assess your medication with your GP, and if appropriate, consultants or paediatricians. I tried to come off everything as soon as I found out I was pregnant, and for 2 weeks I did – however I suffered withdrawals and did not sleep. I eventually got over the withdrawals, and even started to sleep better without sleep medication – possibly due to the pregnancy hormones. In fact I don't think I had slept better since I was a child! But then couldn't function without pain killers – not if I wanted to carry on doing the few hours of work a day that I managed, and to be able to get up the stairs, and do some daily gentle exercise.

The GPs and specialists informed me that the codeine phosphate I was taking was considered safe during pregnancy anyway, so I started to take it again when necessary, but not in the doses I used to. And I was advised to drop the dose or give it up completely in the final weeks of pregnancy, to prevent problems with the baby after birth.

Morning sickness (which should have more accurately been described as 'sickness and/or nausea for any or all of the day whilst you are pregnant) was of course unpleasant, and another symptom to have to go through alongside the increased fatigue and general physical pain of my condition. I did find it hard to cope some days, and took some days off work, but the first time, I didn't have a child to look after yet, so I managed. Thankfully, the nausea only lasted 17 weeks. I know some women have it a lot worse.

I went through my 2nd trimester fairly easily, with just the usual pregnancy symptoms and a bit more back pain.

My existing condition didn't really worsen until the 3rd trimester when I was obviously carrying more weight and walking became increasingly difficult, yet I didn't want to over-medicate. It was not just my back, but hips that were very painful. I did borrow my deceased grandmother's wheelchair for days out or shopping trips, which my husband pushed of course! Another thing that helped was a Dream Genie maternity pillow (for the whole body) and these can often be purchased cheaply on eBay or bought new at Mothercare or online.

Aqua-natal classes in the hydrotherapy pool at my hospital were my best friend. I attended weekly classes and would have gone more frequently if they were available. The day of my class and the day after were my least painful days. Exercising in the cold public swimming pool didn't have the same affect! Anyone with physical pain – pregnant or not, should try and get to a hydrotherapy pool, in my opinion.

I did try the regular aqua fit class in the public pool, but it was too cold and the movements were very jumpy, which made back and hip pain worse. The same applied when not pregnant, but if you can do it without the pain getting worse, it is a great form of exercise. Also I attended weekly prenatal yoga classes, which helped with stretching the hips, keeping good posture, a positive mindset, and relaxing.

As I write I am now in the 2nd trimester of my second pregnancy. Luckily the day long nausea only lasted for 10 weeks. Strangely I experienced a great reduction in back pain during that time, even though I felt sick and exhausted – I can only put this down to the higher level of hormones circulating in the body which must have had a muscle-relaxing effect. When the sickness stopped, the back pain came back with a vengeance.

I wasn't sure how I would fit in these added *'treatments'* and sessions with a consecutive pregnancy, given that I already had another child to care for, but I believe they were extremely important in managing pain, so I am finding ways to access them. I also still had massage to help me during my pregnancy – my therapist customized the treatment for me, and I lay on my side. I am lucky to have a husband who massaged me regularly.

Most mothers will make a birth plan with their midwife, stating what their ideal forms of intervention or alternative ways of coping with the pain of childbirth and delivery will be. I met with a consultant to discuss my options. Since I had previously had a spinal fusion at L4, L5 and S1 (with titanium plates) it was unlikely that an epidural would be effective for me, since it would have to be injected higher up the spine than the usual place. I had elected to have a water birth – knowing the pain relieving effects of warm water for me – so I opted out of the epidural anyway.

Prenatal yoga classes had taught me a lot of positions and massage points that could be used during childbirth, and *'hypnobirthing'* books or classes can also teach a couple some non-medical ways of coping for a more natural birth experience. This includes mindfulness, postures, meditations, etc.. I read a book and watched some YouTube videos about hypnobirthing, but didn't actually pay to attend a course myself, which might have helped more.

Aromatherapy can also be used and is approved by many midwives for use in the delivery suite. I planned a birth that included most of these things, and made a relaxing soundtrack to play in the background. I also had my own TENS machine which was invaluable - these can rented, or be available through your midwife or doula nurse.

Without going into too much detail, in the end, my baby was well overdue, and I had to be medically induced. That resulted in a very fast and strong labour, leaving no time between contractions and I found it quite frightening and hard to cope. There wasn't even time to fill the birthing pool by the time the midwives arrived to deliver him! They put me on my back on the bed, which was probably the most uncomfortable for me (I had thought crouching or kneeling on all fours would have been better). The pain of the contractions was strongest and almost unbearable in my lower back, around my sacrum. With the help of my Mum and husband constantly rubbing this area in circular movements, the TENS machine, and gas and air, we got through it - as women have been since the beginning of humanity.

Of course I was a little more sore than usual for a few weeks after the birth, but painkillers helped, and I later realized that breastfeeding was also providing pain killing endorphins. This was just as well, because the hours I had to sit in a chair trying to breastfeed proved very challenging for me – I never sat still for long even if I wasn't in a lot of pain, but at this time in my life, I had to. I am now past that phase, and my back is no worse. I have to be very careful when lifting my toddler, as it does trigger back pain.

Carrying a baby was a worry for me, but I found the Ergo baby carrier to be a good design for back support, at least until the weight became too much to bear on my hips. Now he can walk, it is easier! But of course now I am considering how I will manage to push two infants, and looking at the lightest weight double prams available.

Purchasing the lightest pushchair possible that is easy to collapse and put up is recommended. For my first child, I went for the Cossatto stroller (from birth) because a travel system would not have been practical for me. We also chose the lightest newborn car seat, but I couldn't carry that for long anyway. Britax make a 360 degree swivel baby car seat, which means you can press a button and it can swivel out to face you when the car door is open, enabling you to lift the child out without twisting as well as bending. From the age of 9 months, MaxiCosi also make a swivel car seat called Axis, which is what I have and it is totally worth the extra cost.

As I prepare for coping with a second baby and toddler, I must admit I am daunted by the physical challenges. But I have a very helpful husband, and will seek out the help I need, as well as any gadgets to help me transport them with the least strain possible.

A cheerful heart is good medicine, but a crushed spirit dries up the bones.

PROVERBS 17:22

SECTION IV

Coping Mentally, Emotionally and Spiritually

CHAPTER 15:

The Neurochemical Link

Our brain chemistry is directly linked with our perception of physical pain, energy levels, and our mood. Treating chronic pain conditions therefore requires a basic understanding of these processes and how we can change our own brain chemistry in order to feel and cope better.

Serotonin is a feel-good neurotransmitter associated with the feelings of relaxation, lessened anxiety, the ability to concentrate, and optimism; serotonin elevates mood and plays a role in fibromyalgia symptoms – especially those with depression and sleep problems. Research indicates that a hypersensitivity to pain, as well as disordered sleep, may in part be due to low levels of serotonin; the lower the serotonin, the lower the pain threshold, and the more disordered the sleep patterns.

Vitamin D is an element that the body also uses to boost serotonin levels, and is best provided by getting out into natural sunlight as often as possible, even if only 2-3 times a week. This is why some people suffer with SAD (Seasonal Affective Disorder) - because of the lack of sunlight during winter months, they can feel 'low' as a result of reduced vitamin D exposure.

Other neurotransmitters help boost attention and energy levels - these are dopamine and norepinephrine – which make us more alert, energetic, assertive and able to concentrate. Tryptophan is an amino acid in the body, which we also convert from proteins in our diet, which is a necessary precursor to the production of dopamine and norepinephrine. Abnormal levels of tryptophan have been observed in some clinical studies of patients with fibromyalgia.

Depression is of course linked with an imbalance of these neurochemicals, as well as being a very common response to living with chronic pain, and is not something to be ashamed of, but treated along with the rest of the physical symptoms. This is one reason why GPs may suggest a prescription of antidepressants to those in chronic pain, another is that these drugs can also have an effect on the system where pain messages are carried through the nervous system to the brain.

Some pain-relieving drugs (such as codeine or tramadol) may even add to feelings of irritability, anxiety, numbness, or hopelessness. I know this can sometimes be the case when I need to take those pain killers.

Here are some factors that can worsen the experience of chronic pain, including some examples of therapies that might be utilised, because these factors need to be managed in a holistic and proactive response to health.

PROBLEM	THINGS THAT MAY HELP MANAGE IT
Anxiety and depression	Medication, CBT, Pain Clinic, group therapy
Fatigue	Treatments for sleep disorders, nutrition
Sleep disturbance	Medication, CBT, exercise, sleep training
Emotional Stress	Counselling, Pain Clinic, social support
Sedentary lifestyle	Appropriate and daily exercise
Physical exhaustion	Pacing (can be learned at Pain Clinic)

STRESS

Simply put, stress is a biological response to demand, that affects the autonomic and central nervous systems. It contributes to illness, depression, back pain, fibromyalgia, and even cancer. Recognizing how your own body and mind show stress is an important step in managing pain - e.g. it could be increased back pain, tension in the neck and shoulders, indigestion, compulsive eating, increased alcohol intake, or lack of creativity and a loss of sense of humour. Managing those symptoms then involves techniques that involve the mind and body - examples of which might be gentle exercise, massage, talking therapies, pacing, and time management. You may need help from a wise friend or a professional, such as a CBT therapist, to help you evaluate the latter three techniques, which might involve planning and setting realistic goals, accepting your limitations, and improving your communication and relationship skills. Attending a program at the pain clinic is also a great option for learning these sorts of management skills.

Exercise is an important tool for managing stress levels - please see my chapter on *Exercise - Movement as Medicine*.

Too much stress can lead to low levels of serotonin and increased levels of cortisol. Cortisol, also known as the stress hormone, is released when we are under any type of stress, and can be helpful to help us take action (the fight, flight or freeze response), but can also be harmful if the stress is sustained or in excess. During periods of increased stress, the immune cells are being bathed in cortisol which tells them to stop fighting, thereby suppressing the immune system and inflammatory pathways, rendering the body more susceptible to disease.

Symptoms of too much cortisol in the body can include things that are often already a problem in those with fibromyalgia and chronic pain, such as:

Severe fatigue

Muscle weakness

Depression, anxiety and irritability

Loss of emotional control

Cognitive difficulties

New or worsened high blood pressure

Headache

Bone loss, leading to fractures over time[37]

So, managing stress is a vital part of learning to manage pain and improve health, and CBT is a tool that can help us learn to do that. The premise of CBT is that our thoughts affect our behavior, which affect the way we feel. Often chronic pain can lead us to think and behave in unhelpful ways and develop bad habits.

---

37. Information derived from http://www.mayoclinic.org/diseases-conditions/cushing-syndrome/symptoms-causes/dxc-20197177

CHAPTER 16:

The Power of Positive Thought

> "You cannot have a positive life and a negative mind"
> *Joyce Meyer*

As explained from the principles of CBT (see section on Pain Clinics), the way we think affects the way we feel. Negative thoughts, for example *"I can't cope, I will never be able to do that, I won't be able to work again..."* etc., will lead to feeling that way physically as well as mentally, and cause us to feel negative emotionally, so we can be on our way down the spiral of depression. Learning to challenge negative thinking with realistic and helpful statements, for example, *"I feel overwhelmed at present, but I can do certain things and get some help to cope with this pain, and tomorrow can be a better day"*, or *" I may need to rest today, but I will feel better later and then tackle that task at an appropriate pace"*.

It is a good idea to attend or join online support groups so that you can have support and understanding from other pain sufferers, then you will also be able to encourage each other as well as be a listening ear, which helps keep your focus not solely on your own troubles. On days when I feel overwhelmed with pain or muscle tension, booking a massage or asking a friend to help massage me, can make me feel less hopeless because I know there is someone to help me, and that I'm very likely to feel much better after a massage.

You may have experienced *'feeling'* better before attending an appointment with a new doctor or therapist who is proposing to offer you some healing - this is because you have hope or belief that something will work, and this can directly affect the way you physically feel. I can testify to this phenomenon, and in some ways it is frustrating because I go to an appointment with apparently a lot less pain than I want them to understand I normally experience!

When I recognize myself thinking - and thus feeling - negative about my condition and my resulting lack of productivity, I find strength in inspiring quotes, books, websites, or scriptures. It can also be helpful to journal at these times - getting thoughts and feelings down on paper that no-one else will see, and somehow then finding my own solutions as I write.

> "The greatest discovery of all time is that a person can change his future by merely changing his attitude."
> *Oprah Winfrey*

> "We can't escape pain; we can't escape the essential nature of our lives. But we do have a choice. We can give in and relent, or we can fight, persevere, and create a life worth living, a noble life. Pain is a fact; our evaluation of it is a choice."
> *Jacob Held*

Please note I am not an advocate of the 19th century New Thought Movement, where God is seen as an all-powerful Mind or Spirit, and man as part of that perfect force. Man only needed to harness the power of this Mind/Spirit to exercise control over illness and the physical world, and therefore, think ourselves healed. This celebration of thinking positively remains engrained in some American culture, as I witnessed whilst living there and seeking healing myself, particularly, and sadly to the excess, in some televangelists and faith healers.

Some interpret the healing scriptures of the Gospels to mean that as good Christians, we are entitled to whatever financial, spiritual and physical health we proclaim over ourselves. I had to practice speaking positive phrases over myself on a daily basis, such as *'I believe I am healed and therefore pain has no place in my body and must be gone in Jesus' name'*. *'I know my back is healed and whole, and I will not accept pain and illnesses'*. These are not bad statements to proclaim and believe in, yet when they were making no physical difference to how my body felt, I began to lose faith. Or I blamed the absent miracle on my own lack of faith, or my own sins. Plus I did not feel I could be honest with people and talk about how I really felt.

'Perhaps you hung onto those pills when Dr Jesus has shown you that you don't need them. Or perhaps you're just not a good enough Christian. Somewhere, somehow, you're to blame[38]'.

I even stopped going to the Healing Rooms because I felt judged and misunderstood, and rarely went up for healing prayer at Church because I was embarrassed every time I was later asked – "Are you healed?" Or "Wow look at the way you walk, hasn't the pain gone and don't you look so much better!'

This attitude is not exclusive to faith healers. I have come across many alternative therapists or so-called *'healers'* who have their roots in other religions and belief systems that also think that we can think ourselves well, and that the universe will rearrange itself to supply what we want.

Having an understanding and acceptance that sometimes, life just sucks, and pain and sickness exist regardless of what we believe, can actually help us maintain our self-respect. *'It can also preserve your overarching happiness by keeping you rooted in reality. The healers will tell you that your pain is subjective: in some cases you have the capacity to suffer less if you think differently about your condition or realize that you don't have to identify with your suffering.... Likewise, if you don't believe you're ever going to amount to anything, then you probably won't; it is worth developing healthy levels of confidence and self-belief if you lack them. Sometimes, focused energy is a very helpful thing, but it doesn't guarantee any results[39]'.* We should learn to make the most of the way things turn out and try to do something positive with what we can.

38. & 39. Derren Brown. Happy. Bantam Press. ©2016 p.49

> 'A cheerful heart is good medicine, but a crushed spirit dries up the bones'.
> *Proverbs 17:22*

Limiting your caffeine intake and paying attention to good nutritional intake can help you manage stress or sleep problems, as well as incorporating relaxation therapies. When you move into a state of relaxation you produce alpha and theta waves in the brain which are consistent with feelings of serenity. Examples of these might be prayer, music therapy, deep breathing, or taking part in arts and crafts.

Beauty

nourishes, balms, & restores the soul.

ART HEALS, SHAUN MCNIFF

CHAPTER 17:

Creativity and Health

There is so much I could say about the benefits of creative therapy – be it through art, dance, crafts, music, or drama. I have been fascinated by the links between the arts and health for many years and at one point was aiming for a career in art therapy. So I know that there are already many books out there explaining in more detail how art (and by that I mean all of the arts) can heal. The focus is generally on the psychological benefits and using arts therapies to treat mental health conditions, but there is also a place for it in treating the physical body and managing painful conditions, such as fibromyalgia, MS, arthritis, or general sufferers of chronic pain. When a natural or medical cure is impossible, there can still be healing therapies and activities available to those suffering. Creative expression through the arts – be in drawing, doodling, painting, crafting, singing, making music, dancing, etc., can be experiences that transport us out of our everyday problems, release our feelings, and lift our spirits.

Art does not profess to rid our afflictions, but to do something constructive with them, to put them to use, so that the feeling of hopelessness or uselessness that can accompany illness is prevented from leading us into depression as well.

I have enjoyed making things with my hands since I was a child. Later, after not really being well enough for full time physical work and failing medical tests to get into nursing or sciences, I studied for an art degree and rediscovered how therapeutic and distracting it can be for me to be immersed in the creative process. Any art studio or art room I have been fortunate to have since, has functioned like a spa – a watering place for my soul.

My final dissertation was based on the use of the arts to treat addictions (having been brought up with parents who run a drug and alcohol rehabilitation centre I had a strong interest in this). Now, I find that creating is an essential part of surviving life and coping with pain, as well as mental or emotional stress.

The application of creative therapies for mental and emotional illness is a much bigger field of practice and fascinating study, based primarily on the concepts of Freudian and Jungian psychotherapy. However, these aspects of ourselves are linked with our physical health as well. Natalie Rogers (daughter of Carl Rogers – one of the main promoters of Humanistic Psychotherapy) explains how symptoms and roots of mental and emotional problems can also affect our physical health:

> 'Repressed thoughts, feelings and behaviours have a lot of power as they rumble around in our unconscious with their potential for volcanic eruption. As with a pressure cooker, the repressed aspects build force by tight containment. Keeping those rumblings in check takes a lot of personal energy. Tension in our muscles, pain in our joints, and constriction of the heart, result from keeping such thoughts and feelings under cover. Most of us fear looking into the unconscious but seldom realise how much physical and emotional energy we spend keeping the lid on.....
>
> Often, however we also relegate to the realm of the unconscious our creativity, strength... so when we risk exploring the depths of the unconscious, we also find many lost treasures[40].'

A lot of chronic pain issues are not sourced in the muscles or areas we can feel it anyway – but actually in your **brain**, when it interprets signals from other parts of your body. **The brain can't concentrate on two compelling activities at the same time, so that's why arts and crafts can literally take our minds off pain.**

---

40. Natalie Rogers. The Creative Connection – Expressive Arts as Healing. ©1993 Science & Behavior Books, Inc p 158

I must mention that when I go to paint – at an allocated time each week because that's all I have and I am trying to be disciplined in my painting practice – this is not always therapeutic. I can get frustrated when I am not able to achieve on canvas what I envision, and get wrapped up in technical difficulty. I often think that what I am doing is inadequate, and become blocked by negative thoughts about the artwork. I put pressure on myself to produce, I self-criticize, and so I do not always find that creative flow that puts me in a meditative and healthier state of mind and body. I have still much to learn in the ability to abandon myself in the painting process. Although I have gone to that therapeutic place at times, especially if not distracted by much physical pain, or with the aid of muscle relaxants - more often I want to experience what Carl Jung describes as,

'often the hands know how to solve a riddle with which the intellect has wrestled in vain[41]'.
Carl Yung

However, with crafts, that have a little more of an instructed process, and when one can see what the outcome should be and have a finished product in sight, I find it a more relaxing and faster-rewarding activity.

I recently started to learn to knit, so that I could make things for my babies but also so that I could have a neat handicraft to do in front of the TV or while listening to music in the evenings, without embarking on a big art project or spreading out my card-making materials all over our living room – as I used to do in my single days! I also wanted a craft I could move around with and do whilst being with other people. I need small portable projects on the go that can be used to manage panic, anxiety, pain spasms and stress or relieve boredom when travelling or trying to 'rest'!

I am finding the technique tricky, and probably tried to run before I could walk by picking complex patterns to follow, and to be honest I find that knitting grows a bit too slowly for me, and I get frustrated when it isn't perfect (which of course it never is because I'm just learning). Yet I keep coming back

---

41. Shaun McNiff. Art Heals. How Creativity Cures the Soul. © 2004 Shambhala Publications p 175

to it - it's addictive! Without realising, I found a new way to really wind-down and relax in the evening, which distracted me from pain, from eating, even from wanting to numb pain by drinking wine! Using crafts, I can subjugate pain to the status of discomfort, so that pain is more of a background feature than an overwhelming stressor.

I simply googled knitting as therapy, and discovered that many others have discovered the health benefits of knitting or crocheting, and in fact knitting groups are being incorporated into pain management programs and hospital groups in the UK. In fact, Betsan Corkhill, a British physiotherapist, founded an organization in Bath (where I am currently based) called Stitchlinks to promote knitting as a therapeutic practice.

Rhythmic repetitive movements seem to put us in the present moment, distracting us from unhelpful past memories or fears of the future. It is a relaxation response and has been found to enhance the release of serotonin, associated with calmness.

If you are trying to manage chronic pain, you probably will have been recommended meditation by well-meaning people, which is nice in theory, but some people are so worked up mentally or uncomfortable physically, that they can't sit still long enough to meditate. That has certainly been my experience, and I have found craft work to be an active, more helpful form of meditation. Of course, most of us have flare up days when pain – especially if in the neck and shoulders or hands, can prevent us really being comfortable doing certain crafty activities. This is why good posture when knitting or making anything is really important. But flare up days sometimes have to be accepted as part of a condition and we may have to 'give in to it' on those days, apply heat, take pain killers or whatever is needed, and instead look at craft books, magazines, or the world of Pinterest to collect ideas and inspiration for days when you can create. I still find these days incredibly frustrating, because I am highly driven and like to be productive all the time, but time for looking, watching and being inspired is also needed in order to create anything.

The internet contains much more evidence from people who have found knitting to help cure their addictions, manage pain, cope with mental illness, and even aid memory for conditions like dementia.

Stitchlinks have a website where you'll find a direct link to researchers and accurate, up-to-date information, ongoing support, information and groups where you can find a community of friends who understand and care. They also produce free practical guides on how to get started with knitting and other handicrafts. With their permission, I have included their list of '25 ways knitting & stitching can help pain' in this book.

Stitchlinks are adding an exciting holistic approach to western medicine:

> 'Our prime focus is on the use of therapeutic knitting as a healthcare tool – unravelling the neuroscience behind its bilateral, cross midline, rhythmic, automatic movements and the complex combination of physiological, psychological, behavioural, social and creative benefits experienced. However, we are also passionate about a 'whole-person' approach to well-being and health care so encourage variety, curiosity, exploration, creativity, laughter and a lot of fun[42]!'

Corkhill sees knitting as a "*constructive addiction*" that can replace other bad habits or addictions. Of course, crochet, cross stitch, and other handicrafts, and especially working with clay, can have the same effects.

> **'In a world where so much of our work is intangible, making things with your palms and fingers gives us a feeling of control and mastery and is way of creating order and beauty[43]'.**

If you have an interest in any creative hobby and want to use it as therapy, then I'm sure you will find a wealth of information online about how that particular activity can help, and encourage you to join a local craft group of that activity so that you can also have the social support, motivation and inspiration from others on days when you really don't feel like doing anything, even if it might be good for you.

---

42. www.stitchlinks.com
43. www.psychologytoday.com/blog/open-gently/201311/should-you-knit

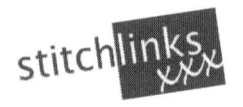

Betsan@stitchlinks.com
www.stitchlinks.com

25 ways knitting and stitching can help pain

- ✓ Facilitate mindful meditation
- ✓ Facilitate relaxation
- ✓ Distract – distraction is one of the most effective analgesics we know of
- ✓ Encourage positive thought cycles helping to break negativity
- ✓ Take pain away from the forefront of your mind
- ✓ Take the focus away from YOU and your pain
- ✓ Motivate you to try other things
- ✓ Improve mood and feelings of depression often associated with pain
- ✓ Improve feelings of loneliness/isolation, giving a sense of belonging
- ✓ Help to manage the stress and worry associated with pain
- ✓ Teach patience and perseverance – help to learn pacing and deal with its frustrations
- ✓ Lessen the frustrations of enforced rest periods – enables productivity at rest
- ✓ Help deal with flare ups
- ✓ Raise self esteem and confidence so you feel better equipped to manage your pain
- ✓ Improve feelings of self worth in society, usefulness and contribution
- ✓ Provide structure and purpose to a day
- ✓ Improve feelings of control for those who feel controlled by their pain, doctors, drugs
- ✓ May break cycles of hyper vigilance to pain
- ✓ Enable you to experience excitement, anticipation and achievement again
- ✓ Help deal with the anticipation of pain by distracting your thoughts away
- ✓ Involve you in the world again – opening up your world
- ✓ Take them anywhere – their portability means you can deal with pain any time, anywhere
- ✓ Calm – dealing with the 'Why me' anger that many feel. Lessening tension
- ✓ Introduce enjoyment and fun into life, so life becomes more than pain and chores
- ✓ Encourage you to look forward to tomorrow

Copyright Stitchlinks   www.stitchlinks.com   November 2007

So when people say about me, *"She never sits still"*, or *"She always has to be doing something"*, it is true. I can't comfortably sit and watch TV or do nothing, without creating with my hands. If I try to, my mind can dwell on the sensations of pain in the body, or things on my mind that might be troubling me. This would normally lead to me trying to numb the pain with more medications, or alcohol, or comfort eating. I am ashamed to say that I also have a long history of bulimia. But by doing crafts, I am distracted from all those negative things and have found a healthy way to cope, and relax, and thoroughly enjoy it!

The field of Art Therapy is huge and fascinating, and thankfully being recognised by even those more scientifically minded as having many benefits to health. Look around the art exhibitions being curated in hospital corridors, as well as art therapy groups running in mental health units and in the community. Not only in the making of art, but by viewing art, can healing be experienced. (For more on how images affect the viewer, read Kandinsky's classic text *'Concerning the Spiritual in Art*'[44]).

Positive visual stimulation has been found to make a difference in the healing process – aesthetic contemplation, i.e. gazing at an object of beauty, can help us get outside of ourselves and become immersed in the object of contemplation, which can revive and refresh us, or give us a feeling of serenity. This is why I find taking a walk in nature – viewing the great Creator's handiwork, or staring at the sky or a sunset, is equally restoring.

If you think drawing or painting is something that might help distract you from pain, there are often groups being advertised and run in your local community centre or library. And an even more accessible and simpler activity that has become very popular recently is adult colouring books, which I also have in my personal toolbox of relaxation techniques.

I haven't mentioned much about music therapy, which is also being explored more now in Western medical establishments as a tool to manage pain. I certainly hope that you have collections of music at home that you put on to help you relax, or energise, or motivate depending on your mood and needs at the time. I have to have music to create, and if I am painting, it usually needs to

---

44. Vassily Kandinsky Concerning the Spiritual in Art, ©1977 Dover Publications Inc. New York.

be classical, but that is down to personal taste. I actually teach piano as my vocation, because it is a job I can fit around daily pain management, family life, and it is not physically demanding. I can be having a really bad day (in terms of pain and fatigue), but once I get immersed in the lesson and focus on the piano student and the music, the pain is displaced more into the background of my awareness.

Music therapy has been proven an effective non-pharmacologic approach to help reduce stress, fear, anxiety, or grief. Some research has found that when used in cases of chronic pain, most patients experienced a higher tolerance for pain; although the level of pain does not change, pleasure, calmness and serenity make it more tolerable. In fact, many of the sensations arising from music and pain are processed in the same part of the brain. Music therapy expert and neurologist Mark Jude Tramo, explains *'We believe music can cause neurochemical changes in specific parts of the brain that are related to the body's feel-good systems—for example, in pain-modulating neurotransmitters. In addition, music's auditory stimulation of the brain may cause cells to release endorphins, which suppress pain, and immunoglobulins, which help fight disease*[45]*'*.

Whilst researching therapies for addictions at a holistic rehabilitation centre in Canada, one of the most powerful sessions I took part in was music therapy which mainly involved drumming – we each had a djembe drum and sat in a circle on a balcony overlooking the beautiful Okanagan Lake in British Columbia. The setting helped aid the creative process of course, but spending two hours working in rhythm and vocals within a group of people all seeking healing, plus a facilitator, put me in a better place mentally, physically and spiritually, releasing tension and negative emotions.

If one is physically able at all to engage in some form of therapeutic dance, this can have a similar effect, but of course most of us are restricted by physical pain. I love to dance, but can only do it with maximum pain killers and then only join in with

---

45. Neurologist Mark Jude Tramo, M.D., Ph.D., director of Harvard's Institute for Music and Brain Science in Boston and a faculty member of the university's Mind/Brain/Behaviour Initiative. http://www.healthcommunities.com/chronic-pain/music-therapy-art-therapy-healing.html

the gentler dances. I do however like to put music on and turn my daily stretching into more of a creative movement session, to make it less boring. If you employ the use of music to aid a relaxation session, it is best to choose a pace of music that is slightly slower than your heart rate, or around 60 beats per minute.

The arts as a whole, can give your brain a break from focusing on the negative.

So I urge you - find a creative outlet, make things, turn your disability or inability to work full time, into something beautiful, and displace the pain for a while.

We are not among those who draw back & perish, but among those who have faith & will possess life.

HEBREWS 10:39

CHAPTER 18:

Spirituality, and Christian Prayer for Healing

Your personal belief system and worldview can have an impact on how you feel emotionally, and that in turn affects your physical health. Achieving inner peace involves coming to terms with our total physical, emotional, mental and spiritual states.

Having a faith may in some cases help people who are suffering, to *'cope better'*. Perhaps it is the belief in a higher Being that can help them or provide them with relief in the afterlife, as well as the moral support of a social group with common beliefs. Connection with other like-minded people is important for the emotional, spiritual, and mental health of any human being, not just those who are suffering.

I am a Christian – a follower of Jesus. It is my belief in a Being greater than myself, who has healing power and strength to impart to me, as well as the future hope of spending eternity in Heaven, where there is no more pain or suffering, that helps me to keep going.

As a Christian, I accept the Biblical teaching on prayer for healing, the laying on of hands, the possibility of miracles, and have sought all of the above for many years. I continue to grapple with certain scriptures over this issue, since I have obviously not received a healing miracle as of yet, and sometimes wonder if I will, this side of Heaven.

I have sought out faith healing, read books about it, attended healing weekends or conferences, visited healing rooms – which is where a group of people lay hands on you and pray specifically for your healing – and done much soul-searching. I have been on inner-healing courses and received Christian counselling, as well as looking at things that might have occurred in my past generations that could have caused my current sickness. I still, frequently ask for prayer from Christian friends or leaders.

I am not yet among the millions of people who have testified to being miraculously healed by God. Yet I don't doubt it is possible and does happen. I don't doubt that He has the power and will to heal those whom He loves. I have seen Him heal my own mother of terminal cancer – completely, without any medical or alternative intervention, only prayer. 20 years later, she is still living, strong and healthy, and we were spared the devastation of losing her.

On my journey I have been healed of emotional pain, and grown to know the scriptures more. I have worshipped with more passion and intimacy. I pray with more desperation. I feel deeply and with empathy for others who are suffering.

I might say I am at peace with God even though I have not been healed, and wait patiently until He does, be that in this life or the next. But to be honest there are days when I do not feel peaceful, I feel cross at my situation and frustrated with my limitations. I get annoyed that I have to spend so much time doing physiotherapy, or resting, or feeling ill from the side effects of medication or ongoing pain and insomnia, when I could be spending that time doing what I thought God had put me here to do – to create things, to paint and draw, to help others.

Ultimately, I have to trust He knows why I have not been healed, and has the grace to give me to endure the pain and frustration, if I will ask for it, and daily depend on Him. I need His grace and wisdom to know how to manage the condition, to pace myself; to know when to fight the pain with medication and exercise, prayer and tenacity of spirit, or to rest. I do not naturally give in to rest and relaxation!

It can be hard to understand why a person isn't healed by God, when He evidently can and does heal people, and Jesus modelled that on earth so often. It should also be acknowledged that sometimes God chooses to work through natural methods or doctors to bring healing.

DOES GOD PROMISE TO HEAL?

We should not assume that because we are Christians, we are exempt from suffering – the Bible in fact tells us to expect it, and why else would we be told to comfort and encourage one another, because *'our destiny is secure in the arms of the Lord, even in the face of suffering and death'*. 1 Thessalonians 4:13 – 5:11.

'We know that the whole creation has been groaning as in the pains of childbirth right up the present time. Not only so, but we ourselves, who have the first fruits of the Spirit, groan inwardly as we wait eagerly for our adoption as sons, the redemption of our bodies. For in this hope we were saved. But hope that is seen is no hope at all. Who hopes for what he already has? But if we hope for what we do not yet have, we wait for it patiently.' Romans 8:22-25 NLT

God never promised us perfect health and the absence of suffering while we are here on earth. The church and those praying for the sick should not act as though He did, for that only causes confusion, frustration, self-condemnation, and even people turning away from their faith.

Many Christians claim that sickness or suffering reflects weakness in a person's faith. I have myself been given this impression many times in the early days of seeking healing through prayer and attending healing rooms and Christian counselling for my condition. However, this view is not founded on scripture. Strong leaders in the Bible, who you would assume had strong faith (as well as the famous example of Job), got sick; and yet Jesus completely healed some who admitted that they had little faith. *'Their depth of faith was not as important as what they put their faith in – Jesus[46]'*.

Jesus taught that we only need faith the size of a mustard seed.

It is also interesting to note that in some cases, those in the Bible who were healed by Jesus had been sick and waiting for a miracle for many years.

In Biblical times in Jerusalem there was a pool named Bethesda,

---

46. Donal O'Mathuna, Ph.D and Walt Larimore, M.D. Alternative Medicine. ©2001 The Christian Handbook. Christian Medical Association Resources and Zondervan Publishing. p.46

which had 5 porches next to it. In these lay multitudes of sick people, waiting for the moving of the water so that they could have a healing miracle. *'For an angel went down at a certain time into the pool and stirred up the water; then whoever stepped in first, after the stirring of the water, was made well of whatever disease he had'.* John 5:4 NKJ

The healing miracle accounted for in John's gospel of one man states that he had an infirmity for 38 years. He would lie waiting for healing at this pool of Bethesda – which Jews would pass by, I presume, each year for an annual feast. Jesus noticed him and healed him completely in this account, but I can't help wonder if there were other years Jesus had attended the annual feast and passed him by – for whatever reason, this was the time the man was healed, and not before. So we cannot know the reasons for God's timing or demand our miracle in a certain time frame or in a certain fashion. Ultimately we have to accept that bad things happen to good people, and we may never know why.

> "For My thoughts are not your thoughts, Nor are your ways My ways," declares the LORD. "For as the heavens are higher than the earth, So are My ways higher than your ways. And My thoughts than your thoughts".
> Isaiah 58:8-9

The teachings and miracles of Jesus show us that God does care for our physical health, and our rest and recovery. So why do bad things happen to good people? Not everyone is healed, and unfortunately many small-minded (though well-meaning) Christians have come up with assumptions on why that may be.

SICKNESS AS CAUSED BY SIN
It is true that sin can result in sickness, or that God allows sickness. In the Old Testament, obedience to God is frequently linked with promises of health and blessing.

Some laws reflect God's concern for his people in choosing natural means to promote health – for example the Israelites were forbidden to eat meat that was likely to carry diseases. The Old Testament clearly teaches that good health depends on obedience to God, and we find that this refers to emotional and spiritual dimensions as well as the physical.

"If you do not obey the Lord your God and do not carefully follow all his commands and decrees I am giving you today... The Lord will plague you with diseases.... with fever and inflammation, with scorching heat and drought, with blight and mildew, which will plague you until you perish". Deut 28:15, 21-22

'I will bring upon you sudden terror, wasting diseases and fever that will destroy your sight and drain away your life'. Leviticus 26:16

When Jesus healed a man, he equated forgiveness with healing, saying *"See you are well again. Stop sinning or something worse may happen to you".* John 5:14. This implies that the man needed to confess his sin and stop it, in order to be healed and continue to walk in health.

The bible teaches that disobedience to God can lead to sickness, which has led some Christians to judge others who are sick as it being caused by their sin, or even that of their ancestors. And in some cases this can be true – a person confesses and deals with their sin, or renounces the sin of their ancestors through the help of something like Sozo Ministries[47], and they are healed.

But after examining oneself and going through healing prayer, confession, and the like, some are still ill. It is common to ask, *"What have I done wrong to deserve this?'* when getting seriously ill or suffering a tragedy. However there is no simple cause and effect relationship between sin and illness. God related to the ancient nation of Israel in significantly different ways than he relates to people today. Israel entered into an agreement with God, where they knew they would be blessed by God if they obeyed him, and swiftly punished by him for disobedience. God

---

47. Sozo Ministries International is a Christian Healing and Deliverance Ministry and UK offering help to people in all forms of spiritual bondage. www.sozo.org.uk

told them, *"See I have set before you today life and prosperity, death and destruction... So choose life in order that you may live, you and your descendants, by loving the LORD your God, by obeying His voice, and by holding fast to Him;..."* Deut 30:15-20.[48]

Today God does not strike people with sickness every time they sin. They might be struck with guilt, which can lead to ill health, which is why we have the offer of God's forgiveness if we confess. This is a free gift from God, not earned by our good works. James emphasises the link between healing and confession:

'Is any of you sick? He should call for the elders of the church to pray over him and anoint him with oil in the name of the Lord. And the prayer offered in faith will make the sick person well; the Lord will raise him up. If he has sinned, he will be forgiven. Therefore confess your sins to each other and pray for each other so that you may be healed. The prayer of a righteous man is powerful and effective'. James 5:14-16

SICKNESS AS CAUSED BY DEMONIC INFLUENCES

The gospels of Matthew and Luke show that sickness can also be caused by demonic influence - in which case, we need not be afraid; prayer can lead to the release of these demon's effects and result in complete healing - Jesus is much more powerful than them! And He who is in us is greater than the one who is in the world.

Some Christians may claim that all sickness has a demonic origin, and therefore the prayer of faith will always heal, and if not, then that person lacks faith. However in the New Testament, clear distinctions are made between illnesses of demonic origin and other causes. Jesus healed people of all kinds of disease and sickness, *'People brought to him all who were ill with various diseases, those suffering severe pain, the demon-possessed, those having seizures, and the paralysed, and he healed them'.* Matthew 4:23-24

Although you may not be sick due to demonic influence, it is important to consider it as a possibility and deal with it as the Bible teaches. Do not think on the other hand that satan's power

---

48. Alternative Medicine. The Christian Handbook. Donal O'Mathuna, Ph.D and Walt Larimore, M.D. Christian Medical Association Resources and Zondervan Publishing. ©2001 p48

over people does not exist, because if you do not believe in the power of satan, you will have no reservation engaging in other spiritual healing practices, and may naively open yourself up to something spiritually harmful.

Artwork, 'Please Heal Me' by Amy Jo Haskins (Samuel). Graphite & Charcoal. 2017 www.amyjo-arts.co.uk

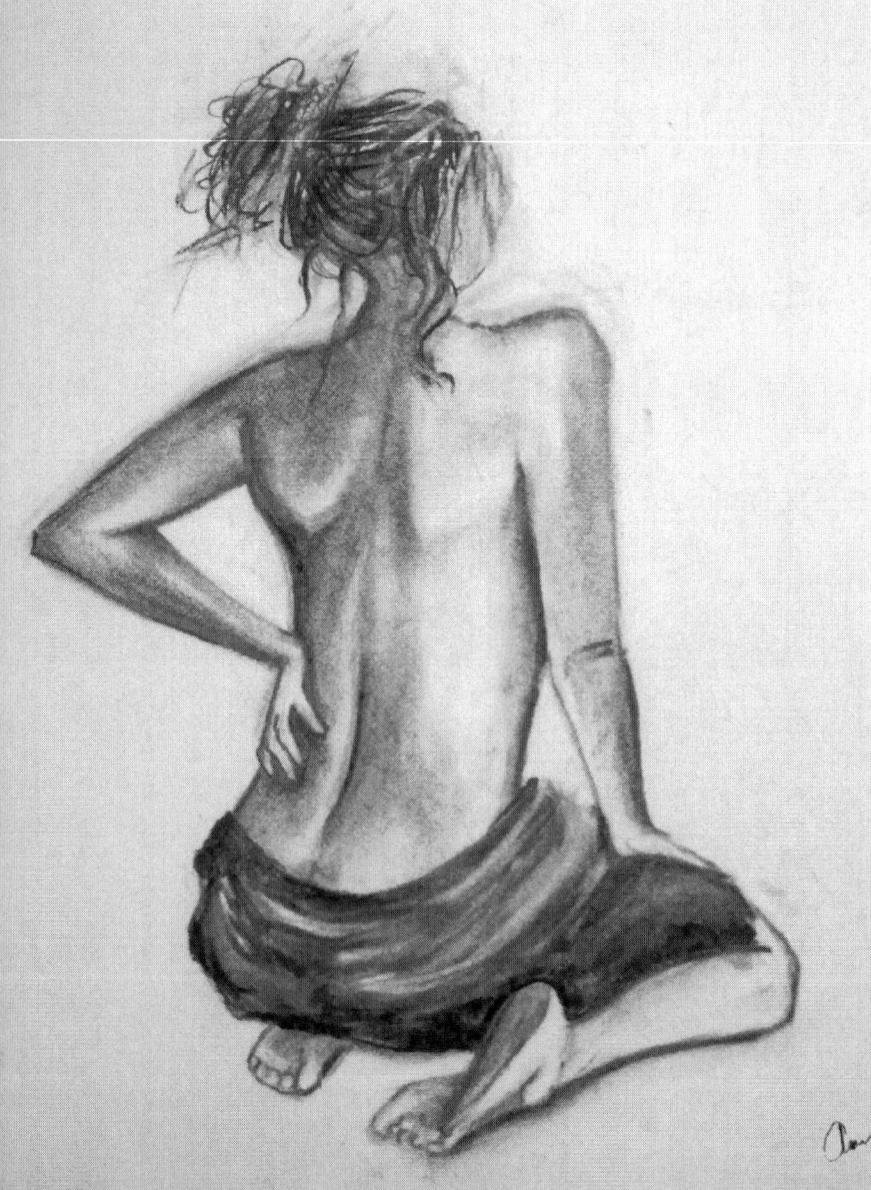

SUMMARY

And after all these points, I believe it is true that some illnesses are purely caused by physical dysfunctions. We live in a fallen world that contains viruses, bacteria, cancers, environmental strains, we may also lead unhealthy lifestyles, and sometimes our bodies break down, don't function properly, and it sucks! Even the Bible accounts for healings where a person was simply just ill, for no apparent reason.

Chronic back pain, fibromyalgia, M.E etc., do not have clear cut causes, and it is hard to accept the fact that we simply do not know the answer. I have come to accept that point (well mostly), and therefore must fully rely on God for the comfort He offers – either directly or through other people, and live the best I can with that, being self disciplined to do all I can do for my health, yet not resenting anyone for the fact that I have not been healed. I also have to ignore the comments of non believing friends and family who say 'If God loved you, why would He allow you to keep suffering in pain?'

I thank God for giving me a husband who knows how to massage to bring relief to me, even though he is not a believer. I thank God for when I have the money to pay for alternative therapies, and for those doctors and physiotherapists that treat me – and of course for the NHS. I believe God's hand has been providing for me all these years through various therapists, friends and family, in order to manage pain, even though I have not been healed. And of course in seeking healing, I was led to many prayer rooms, counselling, and retreats where I experienced much needed inner healing from past issues, and a continued refreshing of God's presence and love.

Although we should pursue physical health, - and in my view especially so that we are released into the calling God has for us so that nothing holds us back - our spiritual health is not to be neglected. When our own physical health is to us of central importance above all else, it can become self-absorbing to the detriment of other aspects of ourselves, our relationships, and spirituality. The belief that we should always be completely healthy and not suffer pain makes it hard to accept illness, limitations, ageing, and loss of a loved one. A lack of health can also lead people to have low self worth and purpose – something I have definitely grappled with over the years that I have been hindered from being as physically productive as I would like. Illness can shake a person's sense of identity if that is dependent on what they 'do' rather than who they are.

As Christians, we know that there is more to life than just physical health, and in all circumstances we should aim to glorify God and serve others, with what we have in our hand and what we are able to do.

My first prayer is that, even having read this book, you may know my Lord and experience a miracle of healing in your body, mind and spirit. My second prayer is that, if you must wait until then, you would glean strength, wisdom and peace from Him, in order to manage your condition well and live in the fullness of life that He desires for you, whatever that may be.

And I will sing like a man, with no sickness in my body.

AS IT IS IN HEAVEN,
HILLSONG 2016

EPILOGUE

For me, managing chronic pain mostly comes down to self discipline - especially with exercising, pacing, and making time to spend doing what I love (creating things), and praying for grace and strength to endure and make something positive and productive with the life I have been given.

I hope that you will not only find healing, but come to know the God who can give you love and grace on your journey.

In all this, if I don't receive healing on this earth, I lookforward to eternity where we are promised a disease-free, tear-free life.

> 'and God will wipe away every tear from their eyes; there shall be no more death, nor sorrow, nor crying. There shall be no more pain, for the former things have passed away.'
>
> *Revelation 21:4 (NKJ)*

BIBLIOGRAPHY

LITERATURE

Brown, Derren. Happy. Bantam Press. ©2016

Donal O'Mathuna, Ph.D and Walt Larimore, M.D. ©2001. Alternative Medicine. The Christian Handbook. Christian Medical Association Resources and Zondervan Publishing.

Dr David Servan-Schrieber. ©2003, 2004, 2005. Healing without Freud or Prozac. Rodale International Publishing.

Dr. Joel Roberston with Tom Monte. © 1997. Natural Prozac – Learning to Release You Body's own Anti-Depressants. HarperCollins

Geddes & Grosset © 2005. Guide to Natural Healing. Geddes & Grosset, Scotland.

Harris H.McIlwain, M.D. and Debra Fulghum Bruce, Ph.D. © 1996. The Fibromyalgia Handbook. Holt Paperbacks. .p 204

Rogers, Natalie. The Creative Connection – Expressive Arts as Healing. ©1993 Science & Behavior Books, Inc

Wassily Kandinsky. ©1977 Concerning the Spiritual in Art. Dover Publications Inc. New York.

WEBSITES

www.name-us.org/defintionspages/DefinitionsArticles/ConsensusDocument%20Overview.pdf

www.verywell.com/causes-of-post-exertional-malaise-716015

www.meassociation.org.uk/2015/10/post-exertional-malaise-in-mecfs-medical-research-council-announces-new-neuroimaging-research-16-october-2015/

Printed in Great Britain
by Amazon